Then There Is No Mountain

"'True story' is an oxymoron."–Butch Hancock

ISBN: 0-6157-4390-0
ISBN-13: 9780615743905

Then There Is No Mountain

An American Memoir

Richard Higgs

TABLE OF CONTENTS

Acknowledgments

Writing is often portrayed as a solitary pursuit. That was not the case in the writing of this book. Thank you Scott Pitcock, Dr. Tom Tomshany, and Laura Frossard for reading the manuscript in its early stages and providing editorial feedback. Your corrections and suggestions were invaluable.

Also, among the many friends who provided material support and encouragement for bringing this book to fruition, I am especially grateful to the following:

Chico & Molly Seay, Barbara Oliver, James Johnson & Rebekah Shields, Dennis & Marian Bires, Walt Kosty & Cynthia Brown, Joe Dennis & Laura Frossard, Scott and Margee Aycock

This book is dedicated to my wife, Louise Joann Higgs

AUTHOR'S NOTE

While writing this memoir, I learned that there's no such thing as a non-fiction narrative.

When you attempt to link events from the chaos of existence into a chain of cause-and-effect, you create a fiction, regardless of your intent, and regardless of your presentation. This is so, whether you're a journalist, a historian, a biographer, a crime-scene witness, a novelist, or a memoirist. Sometimes we present our narratives as nonfiction, but that's just a part of the fiction. Understanding this was very liberating for me.

The stories in this memoir are drawn from both memory and imagination. In these pages, people I know and care about mingle with people who never existed, in places that may or may not be located on any map outside of my imagination. The parts I've drawn from memory, I've drawn as accurately as my memory will allow. But, memory is impressionistic, vague, and subject to change.

A well-told tale is specific, it's rich in sensory detail, and it leads somewhere. Therefore, where my memory left off, I allowed my imagination to fill in the details, so that we both might enjoy the story, and so that the story comes as close as possible to conveying the truth of my experience.

These stories are all fiction, and they are all true.

PROLOGUE

I was sitting in a cloud, breathing with intent. Joe had gone ahead, upward, with the others. Their single-file track in the snow coalesced out of the pale gray gauze a few feet below me and disappeared back into it a few feet above me.

Breathing had become a conscious act, a set of discrete steps. Pull each lungful in through the nose, fill to capacity, hold it for two seconds. Visualize oxygen bubbling into capillaries, and the heart jackhammering enriched bloodfuel down to leg muscles. Force the depleted air out through pursed lips to create backpressure, wringing every molecule. Repeat.

As I sat there on my pack, spine erect, eyes vacant, and my steady breaths adding white to the cloud, a finch, of a type I'd never seen before, appeared and landed on my ski pole sticking out of the snow three feet in front of me. It looked at me hard with first one small dark eye and then the other, and then flicked itself back into the cloud. By my feet, a spider of some kind crept calmly over the pure snow, going through its day. How does it live up here, in the cold, on the snow? When the cold had begun to seep through my layers of mountaineering clothes, I stood up slowly and shouldered my forty-pound pack, ready to continue the climb.

Eric, my patient shepherd, the guide who'd been dispatched to stay with me as I'd fallen further and further behind the team, had been waiting off to the side, watching me. He stood when I did, shouldered his own pack, looked me in the eye, nodded slightly, smiled encouragingly, and together we returned to the trail.

A couple of hours later, when we rejoined the rest of the team in bright sunshine above the clouds at Camp Muir, elevation 10,000 feet and change, they were surprised to see us. They all thought I'd turned back. We'd gotten there about 30 minutes after the last of them. The bright summit of Mount Rainier was still over 4,000 feet above us.

"Where have you all been?" I joked, as they gathered around us. "Eric and I have been worried sick about you. Thank God you're all safe."

Everyone high-fived me, and patted me on the back for not giving up. "Man, am I glad to see you!" Joe said, beaming. He gave me a bro' hug. "They said you'd turned back. Let's get that pack off!" I was glad to see him, too.

Once I'd eaten and rested, and chomped down some chocolate covered coffee beans, Joe and I stood together in the slanting afternoon light, really digging the high, pristine place where we stood. The clouds below us had broken up and drifted away. We looked over what we could see of the path that had led us there. We'd come from Tulsa, Oklahoma, to climb Mount Rainier. We'd crossed many old paths of mine, along the way from Tulsa to Camp Muir.

Except that there's really only one path, and who can say where it begins?

Bigger, Steeper, Colder

Joe and his wife, Laura, had fallen in love with the rarified worlds at higher elevations while climbing in New Mexico's Sangre de Cristo Mountains. They'd climbed Truchas Peak, and they'd climbed Wheeler Peak, the highest point in New Mexico. They'd generously invited me to join them on a subsequent hike up Wheeler, and also, a year later, on a snowshoe ascent up the steep side of Humphreys Peak, the highest point in Arizona. In neither case did I reach the summit. After Humphreys, I was satisfied. I had no further ambitions for climbing anything higher or harder, but Joe had other plans for himself and for me. For Joe, Humphreys Peak had been a skill-building exercise for bigger, steeper, colder mountains to come. Over the next year or so, nearly every time I saw Joe (which was often), he would introduce the subject of Denali. At first it was just facts and figures about Denali. Then it was speculation about what it would be like to climb Denali. Then it was specific information about how long it takes, how much it costs, how one has to train to climb Denali. Then it was speculation about how far ahead we'd need to plan such a climb, how to arrange the time, what our training regimen should be, and what lesser peaks we'd need to bag first.

I fended all this off with noncommittal responses, and tried to change the subject to my own varied preoccupations. "Yeah, Denali, that would be something," I'd say, looking thoughtfully into my coffee cup. And then, "So, what's the deal with viruses, Joe? Are they living or not?" Or, "That sounds like a serious, long-term commitment, Joe," I'd reply, making a show of furrowing my brow, as we walked along his neighborhood streets. "That's a lot of time to block out, Joe. So, anyway, hey, this is a bit off the subject, but what do you think–is information physical? Does it exist outside its container? Or what?" But the pendulum always swung back to climbing Denali.

Eventually, my answers became more pointed: "That sounds like a rich man's sport." "I couldn't get that much time off work." "There's no way I could ever afford that." Joe had an answer for my every answer.

Then There Is No Mountain

Finally, one evening: "Joe, forget it. I'm never climbing Denali. I'm too old, too poor, and too pressed for time. Forget it." After a few weeks of making disparaging remarks about my manhood, and then, finally, dark reminders that life is short and death is long, and that I wasn't getting any younger, he reluctantly dropped the subject of climbing Denali. Our neighborhood strolls, and our idle half-hours at the coffee shop, and our long rambles through the tallgrass once again became occasions for wide-ranging conversations about everything under the sun. But Joe was just biding his time.

I didn't share his burning desire to climb. I was a devoted hiker, not a mountain climber. I was happy, even ecstatic sometimes, just to wade through the lush grasses and wildflowers of Oklahoma's endless rolling prairies. I wouldn't mind dying out there in the grass, some early summer morning, caught in the act of placing one foot in front of the other.

Then, one day in early fall, as the two of us were hiking in the prairie up in the Osage Nation, he said, "Rainier," and it began all over again. I had no intention of climbing Mount Rainier, and told him so, for the same reasons I wasn't going to climb Denali. Too old, too poor, too pressed for time, I said. But as it turned out, after the big scare, I was none of those. I will tell you more later about the big scare.

Candy Creek Ritual

Joe, my wife Louise, and I left Tulsa in the plush sanctum of Joe's big black Land Rover at a little after 6am, headed for Boulder, enroute to climb Mount Rainier in Washington. The tight, familiar, urban weave unraveled to one twisting two-lane threading north out of town, up through the Osage Nation. As we drove along a scruffy oak ridge through the old oil camp of Wolco, we could see across Candy Creek Valley. I pointed out to Louise my old observatory hill sticking up out of the valley, a couple of miles distant. The rubble remains of my old observatory were not visible from where we sat.

When I'd met Louise a dozen or so years earlier, I was a longhaul truck driver, and I'd been on the road long enough that my connections in Tulsa had grown tenuous. I'd been living in the cab of my truck, and all the people I'd once known so well had begun to feel remote to me. Truck driving will do that to you after a while. You spend all your time on the road either completely alone or in the company of strangers you'll never see again. I no longer had a place to stay in Tulsa, or at least it felt that way. By the time I quit trucking, I'd been seeing Louise whenever I'd pass through town, but staying at her place was out of the question, so I'd been sleeping in the truck when I stopped in Tulsa, just like I did in any other city. So, when I parked my truck in the Oklahoma City truckyard one July morning, and drew my pay for the last time, and drove my beloved old Saab back to Tulsa, my first stop was an army surplus store.

I bought a sleeping bag, mosquito netting, insect repellent, a coffee percolator, some galvanized plates and cups, a couple of lightweight tarps, a backpack, and other supplies, including a very cool pith helmet (the only hat I've ever looked good in, although Louise has a different opinion about this). Then I stopped at a liquor store and got a pint of W. L. Weller bourbon. Lastly, I stopped at Walmart and bought a rod and reel and some tackle. Then I drove up north, past the town of Skiatook to Candy Creek.

Then There Is No Mountain

Candy Creek has wallowed out a wild valley from the prairies of the old Osage Nation. Over the years, I've hiked every one of the valley's 25 miles or so, and fished much of the creek, from its source to its mouth, through the wild horse pastures in the upper end, down into the broader, partially wooded lower end where it feeds into Bird Creek. Candy Creek Valley formed the back pastures for a series of large ranches along its course, so virtually no one lived in it. The lower end had been bought out by the Corps of Engineers for a dam project. The project was abandoned while still on the drawing boards. Once this happened, the valley became orphaned land–owned by the public, but managed by no one. It had always been wild, but in its abandonment, it began actively returning to an earlier, wilder state.

I knew of some limestone springs that never went dry, out there deep in the valley. The water was cool and sweet. I drove as far as I could down the abandoned valley road, hid my car behind a sand plum thicket, and then hiked to the springs with my gear. The first thing I did was dip my cup into the spring and drink, again and again, until I could feel the water's weight in my belly. I spent the hot, humid July afternoon setting up a lean-to camp in the deep shade near one of the springs. I caught a couple of bass out of Candy Creek which I filleted, wrapped in foil, and cooked in the coals of my small fire, next to the chiming streamlet that tumbled out of the stone.

As the sun went down I sprayed myself with mosquito repellent, arranged my small fire so that I'd have something to look at as it slowly burned down, and sipped on Weller's and spring water from my tin cup.

"You need to make a plan," I said to myself. "Yeah, but not right now," I replied.

Summer nights in the wild tanglevine Oklahoma bottomland are noisy. All around me, near and far, all the creatures of the world, it seemed, howled, bellowed and screamed all night long. Packs of coyotes on the move howled back and forth to each other, cattle bellowed on the distant upland pastures, dogs on the hunt yelped for joy, hoot owls and whippoorwills sang to themselves, frogs rang together like a thousand stuck doorbells, and countless unknowable species of insects created a conglomerate pulsing high-pitched drone. There was also the annoying, recurring whine of mosquitoes probing around me for a way past the DEET.

The Weller's and the campfire diminished at about the same rate. By the time the bottle was empty and the fire was out, I'd added my own voice to the chorus. The first time I howled, every other creature stopped to listen. After about thirty seconds, the insects could stand the silence no more and started up again, quickly rejoined by the frogs, and then all the others. The second time I howled, they all quieted down just for a moment and then carried on. The third time I howled, my voice just blended in.

In the bright morning sunlight, I set the coffeepot off the fire, it stopped perking, and I could once again hear the little stream tumbling away from the limestone spring. I poured a cup of coffee and sat with it in my hands, looking at the blue smoke rising like a genie. "You know what your problem is?" I asked myself.

"No, but I have a feeling you're going to tell me," I replied.

"You need more ritual in your life." As a truck driver, I'd been living as a human pinball, bouncing randomly all over America, never knowing what direction or how far I'd bounce next. I thought about that for a while as I drank my coffee.

"Maybe you're right," I replied, once I'd emptied my cup and stood up to break camp. "And I still need a plan, too," I said. Well, my plan was simplicity itself. I packed out, drove the old Saab to Tulsa, got an apartment by noon, and a job by the next day. Louise and I married and bought a house, and she and I and her son, Robin, whom I came to call my own son, moved into the house, and then he grew up and moved out. Then it was just the two of us in our small home, which we'd filled with books, music, and art. Much of the art is of her own creation. She is a brilliant and passionate painter.

Although I lived there, so to speak, only for one night, I remained, over the years, a frequent visitor to Candy Creek. Sometimes, I stayed close to the creek and fished the deep holes. Sometimes, I rambled the meadows, glassing birds, and sometimes I just walked, exploring the rocky sidestreams that tumbled down from the surrounding uplands. Sometimes, I mused about the lack of ritual in my life. I wondered what it was like to take comfort in ritual. If you perform an act over and over again, an act that may otherwise be meaningless—that would almost certainly be meaningless if done only once—and you perform it in the same way each time, and at specified intervals, what do you get from that? Why is that attention to form so comforting to so many, so central to their self-identities? I felt I must be missing out on something.

One day out there, I looked across the valley from the eastern ridge and noticed on the opposite ridge, about three miles distant, an isolated knob, a little higher than the surrounding terrain. It had a pleasing curve and a copse of blackjack oaks on the crown. As I dropped down into the valley, it disappeared from view, so I walked across the valley floor, and then up the opposite hill, sensing my way toward it by dead reckoning, until it re-emerged above me. Before long, I was standing on top of it. Just as I'd known I would, I had a clear view of the distant horizon in all directions. Looking east over the valley to the opposite ridgeline, from where I'd come, I decided to build an observatory on the spot, where I could witness the sunrise on the first day of spring and the first day of autumn every year. I would make it a ritual, and see what came of it.

I stacked fieldstones, ruddy sandstones, into a cairn about a foot taller than myself. At eye-level I left a window, about six inches square, that passed through the stones as a viewfinder. In the base of the window I placed a flat stone that protruded out from the cairn and came to a point which pointed due east, according to my compass. In the stone I cut a groove in a straight line as a sightline which ended at the point. Standing up to the cairn on its west side and looking into the viewfinder and following the sightline groove, my eye landed on the spot on the far horizon where the sun should pop up on the vernal and autumnal equinoxes.

I admired my observatory from various distances as I hiked the several miles back to my car. Its form and function were pleasingly mysterious. Once the grass had covered my footsteps around its base, and healed the scars where the stones had been removed, it would be difficult for anyone to know how old it was, which also pleased me.

I awaited the first day of fall with growing anticipation. I took three days off from work. The day before, I packed up and went out there. I found a pretty site in the edge of the woods at the base of the observatory hill and set up camp in the afternoon. I built a hearth and a lean-to and gathered firewood. Then I searched among boulders in a shady draw until I found the right one and, using a chisel and hammer, I cut an image of a horse into its side. I'd stolen the design from a centuries-old Chinese drawing. I returned to camp and got a fire going. I heated up some beans and made coffee. After supper I climbed up to the top of the observatory hill. First I inspected the observatory, but avoided looking through the viewfinder. It was unchanged in the months since I'd erected it. Then I found a good place to sit and faced west, where I watched the sun lower itself down to the horizon and melt like butter on a griddle. Once the first star came out, I walked back down to camp. I stared into the fire for a while. There was nothing on my mind. Then I stared up at the Milky Way for a while, and scanned it with my binoculars, not looking for anything but beauty, which was there aplenty. I didn't have a watch, but I imagined it was still pretty early when I crawled into my sleeping bag and fell asleep.

When I woke up it was cold, and deep dark. The Big Dipper had spun around the sky. I stoked up the fire and fell back asleep. When I woke again it was still dark, but it felt like morning inside me. I dressed, banked up the coals in the hearth and put on coffee. While the coffee perked I was alert to the changing light of the sky. I was getting excited. I would have hated oversleeping—and missing my first observation. I took my coffee and drank it standing out from under the trees, in the chilly wind, watching the sky closely as the stars dimmed.

I climbed to the top of the hill and stood around the observatory watching the eastern horizon. I felt more like a kid at Christmas than a man in September. The sky grew lighter and lighter until finally the sun was seconds away from rising. I took my position and looked down the sightline and waited. There he was! My sightline was off a couple of degrees, so I quickly adjusted it with a couple of nudges. It was now empirically correct. Once the sun had cleared the earth I stepped back from the viewfinder, having completed my first observation.

I felt as if I hadn't merely witnessed the turning of the earth, and swinging of the seasons, but that I had actively participated in these. After savoring the experience for a good long while, I went back down the hill to camp and had a leisurely breakfast in the crisp fall sunshine. Over breakfast, I pondered how the sunrise swings back and forth along the horizon between the spring and fall equinoxes. It behaves like a pendulum.

A pendulum's speed varies constantly during its stroke, reaches maximum velocity at the bottom, and slows to a stop at each turnaround point, before reversing direction and accelerating back to the bottom. The sun's apparent speed (as measured by its changing day-to-day position on the horizon, as it swings out the seasons) also varies constantly, and in the same manner. Around the equinoxes, the sunrise positions change most rapidly. Approaching the solstices, the position changes slow to a stop, reverse direction and begin accelerating back to the next equinox.

Why should the sun behave like a pendulum? It seems like a clue to something.

I spent the day exploring the woods and prairies around me. Just before sunset, I climbed back up the hill and observed the sunset looking back through the viewfinder from the opposite side. I spent another night in camp, and the next morning I broke camp after breakfast and walked down the valley to my waiting car. I got back to Tulsa mid-afternoon.

That became my twice-a-year ritual for the next several years. Hike up to my camp the day before, spend the night, observe the sunrise, spend the day lounging, hiking around, and pecking images into the boulders, then spend another night, and hike out the next day. It was important to seal off a full 24-hour period on-site, in order to fully inhabit the place. I remember waiting atop the hill near the observatory, in the chilly pre-dawn, sometimes wrapped in a blanket, sipping coffee, my heart pounding, and my smoke-stung eyes riveted on the horizon beyond the valley as the sky grew lighter and lighter. I remember a feeling of victory as the top rim of the sun shimmered into view right at the end of my viewfinder sightline.

Did I gain meaning from this ritual? Leading up to each spring and fall season, as the pivotal day grew closer on the calendar, I became more and more restless in the city. By the time I headed out, I'd been thinking of little else for several days. When I came back from out there, I felt satisfied and serene for days afterward, so it seemed as if I'd found what I was missing out on.

One late afternoon out there I looked up at the hill from the edge of the woods by my camp and saw that one of the hilltop oaks was on fire. Looking more closely, I saw that it wasn't really aflame but was glowing strangely, unlike any of the trees around it. Unlike anything I'd ever seen. I climbed up there to see what was going on. To my wonder, I discovered that it was covered with monarch butterflies, as thick as leaves. There were thousands of them, all basking in the late afternoon sunlight. They'd stopped to spend the night during their migration to Mexico. I laughed out loud, and thanked God for letting me see such a sight.

After several seasons of not allowing anything to get in the way of my semi-annual three-day ritual, one spring, I let something stop me from going. I don't recall what it was. My usual feelings of mounting excitement and restlessness had been muted that year. I witnessed the equinox sunrise from the driver's seat of my car on my way to work. I couldn't have missed it, actually, since Tulsa's streets are a cardinal grid, and the sun rose right out at the end of the street, blinding all eastbound drivers. I'd be willing to bet that auto accident records for Tulsa would show a spike on the equinoxes.

I was disappointed in myself, so the following fall, I made sure to set everything else aside and went out to the observatory. I had a fine time, as always, but my observation felt rote, my emotional involvement felt forced. The following spring was about the same. I missed the following fall and subsequent spring.

Then There Is No Mountain

I went out one last time the following fall, but the spell had been broken. I sat on the hill and thought about it. I realized that I'd put the cart before the horse by trying to manufacture meaning out of ritual. Rituals arise out of pre-existing meaning. They *confirm* something meaningful. That's what I learned about the power of rituals. Since then, I've returned to my old ritual-free way of life. I claim no credit for the fact that the sun still rises at the same spot on the horizon every spring and fall equinox.

Although I continued to occasionally hike, fish, and camp in Candy Creek Valley, it was several years before I trekked back up to my observatory hill to visit. I was surprised to find that my cairn had collapsed into a random pile of rubble. I blamed it on cows, those dumb agents of entropy. The only remaining signs of my having been there were the crude hearth at my old campsite, and the images I'd pecked into certain boulders.

Tulsa to Boulder

On we rolled–Joe, Louise, and I—through the tallgrass prairies of the Osage, prairies once again grazed by bison, and wild horses in the thousands. The grass waved us forward in the wind like a wildly cheering crowd. We rolled westward, through Ponca City, then turned onto I-35 north. The monoculture-and-feedlot wasteland of western Kansas consumed the rest of the morning and much of the afternoon under a blue enameled sky. Somewhere out there, in the wind between Grinnel and Colby, we crossed an old path of mine. I'd once worked the wheat harvest out there (which I've written about in my book *Bringing In The Sheaves*.)

Past the Kansas-Colorado border (the last frontier, the once and future buffalo commons), the irrigation farming, made possible by the ever-diminishing Ogallala aquifer, plays out to the shortgrass plains of Eastern Colorado. As we drove on, Pronghorn Antelope loafed by the side of the road. I've always wanted to taste antelope. Pike's Peak came into view, then Denver at rush hour. Miraculously, we slipped right through Denver, ricocheting off the city's northeast side and rocketing on to Boulder, as traffic backed up four lanes wide and miles deep on the other side of the median. We found our Best Western motel in Boulder easily, checked in, freshened up and drove downtown to the mall to check out the streetlife and have dinner at The Kitchen. I gaped at the amazing Flatirons, just south of town. Enormous slabs of sedimentary strata hinge upward at an extreme angle, at the very western end of the Great Plains, like a trapdoor, up through which rises the Front Range of the Rocky Mountains.

Enlightened Boulder is, in addition to its university population, a magnet for vagabonds, panhandlers, buskers, jugglers, moneyed hipsters, vegetarian singles, mountain hikers, and bikers, and they were all there strolling the promenade that mild summer night. We had a 30-minute wait for a table at The Kitchen. They took Louise's cell number to call when one became available. We had a drink while we waited, in a nerve-wrackingly loud bar next door. Packs of twenty-somethings yelled happily at each other over the pounding music, sharing iced buckets of Bud Light. It was difficult to tell the waitstaff from the customers, but we flagged down a server. We didn't have the energy to yell at each other, so we quietly nursed our beers until Louise's phone rang.

The meal at The Kitchen was a treat. I had lamb from a local farm, and we all had salads that seem to have been picked about three minutes before reaching our mouths, along with good wine, dessert, and a shared glass of tawny port. A satisfying end to a long day on the road. Joe generously picked up the enormous tab. Louise and I exchanged glances but didn't protest.

On the quiet ride back to the motel, sated and sentimental, I mused over Joe's loyalty and generosity. When I'd pled poverty as a reason I couldn't go climb Mount Rainier with him, he'd offered to pay most of our expenses. "Money is just a tool," he said. "I happen to have more access to it right now. We're a team, you and me, a climbing team, so we each do for the team what we can." Still, picking up the tab at The Kitchen was above and beyond.

While I was in the hospital the previous summer, nearly every time I woke up, Joe had been there, watching out for me. I remember him fending off my delusional alcoholic roommate and his swarming cloud of staph germs as the guy reeled around the room, shouting incoherently, his rolling IV stand careening in tow. And just a couple of weeks before our meal at The Kitchen, when Louise had taken me to an emergency room in Tulsa, Joe had met us there, and sat with us in the woeful waiting room until we gave up and went home.

The Beggars of Boulder

At the Best Western, I woke up early, about 5:30, slipped into running shorts, quietly to not wake Louise, and went for a run on the gray-dawn empty streets. I ran south a few blocks to Boulder Creek, then along the creek, thinking how lucky they were to have a mountain stream coursing through the heart of their city. I was running to catch up. A couple of weeks before, just when I'd meant to kick the aerobic part of my pre-climb training into a higher gear, I'd found myself doubled over with severe abdominal pain. The pain lasted, intermittently, for 3 days, before I went to the doctor. He prescribed some anti-spasmodic pills, telling me to let him know if it wasn't better in a week. By the next night I was rocking back and forth holding my gut in the St. John's emergency room with Louise and Joe in attendance. Hours went by, and the nurses never called my name. About midnight the pain subsided enough that we just went back home. I took a sleeping pill. Next morning I went back to the doctor. He gave me another prescription for a powerful painkiller and told me, "The anti-spasmodic needs to build up in your system for a few days before it can work." If I had no improvement in a few days, he'd order an ultrasound of my gallbladder. "Doc, I'm leaving to climb Mt. Rainier at the end of next week. I need to know ASAP if my gallbladder's gone bad." He scheduled the ultrasound for the earliest date possible, midweek the following week. By that date—two days before we were to hit the road—the pain had disappeared, and the ultrasound concluded that my innards were "grossly unremarkable", according to the report. I was cleared to climb, but my training routine had been brought to a halt at a crucial time, so my conditioning had lost ground instead of gaining. The mysterious pain was never explained. I was running to catch up, and I ran hard, that morning in Boulder.

We'd planned to have breakfast in Boulder and then drive up to Rocky Mountain National Park, to the Alpine Visitor Center, which would take us to about 12,000 feet. That would be our only opportunity to acclimate to high altitude before climbing Rainier. *My* agenda was to have a quick breakfast and start driving, to spend as much of our day as possible up there. I stopped at a coffee shop, just opening, on the way back to the motel, got Louise and myself coffees, and carried them to the room. I saw Joe in the motel parking lot and told him about the coffee shop, a couple of blocks away. "I wonder if they have wi-fi," he replied. I told him that I'd noticed that they did, so he headed that way with his laptop.

A few minutes later, Louise and I drove the Rover to the coffee shop to pick Joe up for breakfast. "Joe," I said, "I was thinking we need to get up to the mountains as early as we can so we can spend as much time as possible at altitude today, enjoy the scenery, Louise can sketch, and we can get back down before the afternoon storms begin up there. So why don't we just have breakfast just any old place that's quick, and get rollin'? There's an IHOP about a block from here."

"IHOP? We can eat at IHOP anywhere." Joe seemed to be in a bad mood.

"Well, what do you want to do?"

"Well, I don't want to eat at IHOP." He folded up his laptop.

"Okay, then, what?"

"There's gotta be a place back down on the mall that serves breakfast." We walked to the Rover.

"Well, I just didn't want to make a big production out of trying to navigate around, getting frustrated, expending a lot of time and effort looking for just the right place. I want to get up to the mountains."

"We'll find someplace."

I shrugged, and sighed inside. "Lead on, then."

Joe climbed into the driver's seat. "Which way to the mall?"

I sighed again. This time on the outside. "It's the same route we took last night. Make two rights and a left, go all the way down to 14th, make two rights and that will get us back to that parking garage." A few minutes later, after only a couple of wrong turns, we got parked. I led us out of the garage and onto the mall. The three of us stood in a group, each waiting for the other to lead. Feeling a bit passive-aggressive, I was determined to follow as we searched the mall for breakfast, so when Joe looked at me, I just gave him a dumb look. If it had been up to me, we'd have been finishing the last of our pancakes about then, and just about to head to the mountains. Joe took the lead, and to his credit, within two blocks, found a place open for breakfast, which we enjoyed on the patio, people-watching as we ate. Louise ordered more than she could eat, and once she'd finished, she asked for a to-go box. I tried to dissuade her because breakfast doesn't travel well. When did she plan to eat it? She refused to be dissuaded, so she carried her breakfast leftovers as we strolled along the mall back toward the Land Rover. Joe wanted to browse in a bookstore. I looked at my watch. Morning was waning. "What about the mountains?" I asked, so he dropped it.

A skinny young panhandler in tatters approached us and, eyeing Louise's to-go box, boldly asked if he could have our leftovers. Joe, who has studied martial arts, spun toward him with ninja-swiftness and planted his feet, shielding Louise and me. "No," said Joe, fixing the boy with a look of fire and ice. The beggar stepped back. Louise's eyes met mine. "I could," she said. "You should," I replied. We both knew she'd never eat it. Maybe this was why she'd felt compelled to keep it, without knowing it. I called the beggar back, over Joe's shoulder. He arced around Joe to get within reach of us. Louise handed the food to me, and I handed the food to him. He thanked us and told Louise that she was a very nice person. "And you are rude!" he said to Joe, once he had secure possession of the food, and had backed away several feet. "You're a rude person!" "No, he's not," I called back. "He's a good guy. Just go on, now. Enjoy it."

Joe seemed abashed as we continued. "I guess I need to work on being more laid-back in Boulder," he said. He'd also been called rude the night before by an intoxicated young woman seated next to him in the bar where we'd waited for our table at The Kitchen. She'd tried to strike up a conversation and he'd brushed her off, thinking, as he told us later: "Look, I'm 54 years old, married and sober. You're 24, drunk, and I-don't-know-what. I don't want to talk to you. We have nothing to say to each other. Just don't talk to me." He'd conveyed all this to her with his fire-and-ice look. She'd told him he was rude and turned back to her friends.

I felt bad for him. "Ah, you're okay. Don't sweat it."

"I'm like a bull in a china shop in this town. Which way is the truck?"

Next to the motel was an REI store that we'd previously spotted. REI is the ultimate department store for outdoor adventurers.

"Let's stop in there for a minute before we head up to the mountains," Joe suggested. "I want to look at their boots."

"The morning's wasting, Joe," I replied. In our many planning sessions over the last few months, spending the day in the mountains, after we'd awoken in Boulder, was part of the plan. We'd agreed on it, and we'd agreed on the reason why–acclimation. Still, I needed a base layer of clothing for our climb, and we were right outside the store.

"We can take a few minutes," he replied. "The mountains will still be there."

I really did need to get a base layer of clothing for the climb. "And then we head out. Right?"

"Right."

We parked in front of the store. Louise walked over to the motel to wait while we shopped.

Once we were inside the store -a bustling wonderland of outdoor clothing, accessories, equipment, and supplies- Joe and I quickly separated. As I winnowed through the smart crowds of relentlessly fit, impeccably dressed shoppers, I lost all sense of time. Layers of polyester and wool accumulated over my left forearm.

I found Joe in the boot department, trying on mountaineering boots. He had four different brands piled around him as he tried on a fifth pair. The store had set up an inclined plane for testing. He laced up the boots, and then thoughtfully climbed up and down in them several times. He sat on the low bench, looking vexed. "I just can't decide," he said. I drifted away.

Joe found me later in the close-out department. I was squeezing between parkas stuffed together on a rack, to get to another rack behind it. When he said my name, I spun around and got caught up for a moment in the parkas. Once I'd extricated myself, and my purchases, and we stood facing each other, Joe asked me what time it was. I looked at my watch.

"Holy crap! We've been in here for an hour and a half!"

"Oops. Let's get going."

We checked out, picked up Louise, and got on the road, feeling sheepish about squandering our morning. Joe, I noticed, never did buy any boots.

When we arrived at Estes Park we stopped for a joyless lunch at the Stanley Hotel, in the dimly lit, shopworn dining room. The service was indifferent, the food was overpriced, and the menu featured novelty meats. I had an elk burger. Anonymous red meat. Once we finally found someone willing to take payment, we left and headed up to the high country. By then, the afternoon rains had begun, as we'd known they would, as they do daily on summer afternoons in the mountains. Joe, at the wheel, became freaked out by the wet road, and the sheer drops and switchbacks. Holding the steering wheel in a deathgrip, not looking left or right, he began to straddle the yellow line between the two lanes. Those descending, on the other side of the road, just had to find what room they could to get around us. A parade began to form behind us. At a little above 10,000 feet there was an overlook turnout, which we pulled into. We all jumped out, glad to be stationary and out of the tension-filled vehicle. There wasn't much view due to the cloud cover and rain, so after using the facilities and then walking around a little to stretch, we sat in the car for a few minutes and breathed with intent. Joe refused to go any higher, even with me driving, and I didn't push the point. It was raining up there, anyway. "I have no trouble walking or climbing in high, steep places, but in a vehicle, it's just——," he finished with a shudder.

I drove us back down at what was a comfortable speed for me, but both Joe and Louise kept gasping for me to slow down. They pressed imaginary brake pedals going in to the curves. Eventually I slowed to a speed they found comfortable, and we led another parade of cars back down the mountain. Our excursion to Rocky Mountain National Park had been kind of a bust.

As we neared Boulder, Joe suggested we browse that bookstore he'd seen on the mall, which sounded okay to me. It was something to do with the evening. Something in the way he said it caused Louise to believe that he meant to exclude her. She became highly offended, unbeknownst to me, so that when Joe asked her if she thought that would be fun, she declined to participate. It was obvious to her that he didn't want her along. Since it would only be Joe and me, I suggested an urban hike from our motel to the bookstore. She then became convinced that both Joe and I wanted to exclude her, since she's not one for hiking. I was oblivious to how Louise was feeling about all this, and was caught by surprise when she laid it all out for me, privately, a few minutes later in our room. I'd thought she'd declined to join our excursion to the bookstore so she could have some time alone. I was indifferent to whether she came along with us or not, and told her so, which only made her angrier. Which made me angry, so I left in a huff.

Boulder to Rock Springs

I got up early and took another run in gray light along Boulder's deserted streets. Louise suggested we breakfast at Lucille's, a Cajun-style restaurant in an old Victorian house downtown. We got there 30 minutes before they opened. It was Father's Day, and there were already three or four families in line. There were tables set up on the front porch, and it was a sweet morning, so I suggested to Joe and Louise that one of those tables would be nice. Louise nodded silently, but Joe didn't seem to like the idea.

"I don't know about that," he said, creasing his brow. "I don't think so." He seemed to be pondering a private objection.

"Why?" I asked.

"Oh, I don't know," he replied, shaking his head. He looked as though his objection came from some deep place that couldn't be explained.

Once they opened and began seating people, it was clear that there would be a lot of foot traffic, in and out on the porch, so as we made our way to the host to be seated, I told Joe I thought he was right. We should sit inside after all.

"No, let's sit outside," Joe said.

"Too much traffic," I countered.

"No, it isn't," he argued. We were standing at the host's station. The host looked expectantly at me. Annoyed by Joe's contrariness, I shrugged and asked for a table on the porch.

As we were taking our seats, I was glad Joe had insisted, but then he said, "Oh, I don't know about this. This doesn't feel right." I shot him a warning look to drop it, which he did. Louise had remained silent during all of this. Our breakfast was so amazingly good, and the morning so fine, it chased away all the tension and confusion.

It was decided that I should drive the first leg on our long drive to Twin Falls, Idaho, with Joe navigating. About two blocks from the motel, we missed a turn. We'd driven in the wrong direction for about twenty minutes before we realized the error, so we backtracked to Boulder, found our turn, and headed east toward I-25 northbound. As the shining Flatirons diminished in our rearview mirrors, it occurred to me that things hadn't gone very well in Boulder.

When we got to Cheyenne, Wyoming we turned west onto I-80 and the wild, windswept, high plains of Wyoming. Our route kept us mostly above 7,000 feet all the way across the state, the exceptions being where we dipped down into the few riverside settlements along the way. It had evidently been a wet spring because the short grass plains were vivid green to the horizon. The Medicine Bow Mountains, the Green Mountains, the Wind River Mountains, all rose above distant horizons and slowly lowered again as we sped west. We stopped and switched drivers at some nameless place in the wind.

At Rawlins we stopped at the McDonald's, entering through the exit, and after a laborious U-turn, got in line at the drive-thru. The attendant's timid voice coming over the speaker was all but drowned out by the bawling sound of a herd of highly agitated cows, also coming over the speaker. We looked at each other in puzzlement. What the hell was going on in there? After having to repeat it a couple of times, we got our order placed and pulled around to pick it up. There the mystery was explained. A cattle truck was parked on the other side of the building and the cattle were (understandably) in a state of high anxiety, howling and kicking at the sides of the trailer as their driver sat inside eating you-know-what. True to form, we exited through the entrance, then turned left, when we should have turned right, did a U-turn, and got back onto I-80 west.

Just past Rawlins, we crossed the Continental Divide, the *Great* Divide, a place I'd been watching for. If you want to understand the lay of the land, you have to know how the waters flow. For me, waters flowing into the Pacific Ocean provide the most fundamental definition of The American West. However, despite having crossed the Great Divide, we weren't quite there yet.

The river systems that drain and define continental topographies are well-known, because water equals life and locomotion. Rivers and their tributaries are named, mapped, and storied. Less familiar is the system of divides that separate and fold around those watersheds. The two systems form an infinitely complex, recursive jigsaw puzzle with only two pieces: watersheds and divides. All watersheds large and small drain from an ultimately common line—the Continental Divide—and spiral out from that line. They converge, as they drop, into rivers that terminate at far-flung points on a common plane—the ocean. All divides large and small rise from far-flung points along that same plane, converging as they *rise* to terminate ultimately along a common line—the Continental Divide. From line to plane, from plane to line, the two systems create and define each other. Together, they comprise a continent's topography. You can walk down a watershed from the top of Isolation Peak in Colorado to the Pacific's Sea of Cortez, or down a different watershed from that same mountain to the Atlantic's Gulf of Mexico. You could also, in theory, walk along converging ridgelines from the ocean back to the top of Isolation Peak.

Places can form in continents which aren't part of the great drainage system, however. As we crossed the divide west of Rawlins, we entered such a place. The Continental Divide splits at Continental Peak in the north and rejoins at Separation Peak in the south. The loop thus formed is called the Great Divide Basin. Interstate 80 cuts across the southern part of this basin for about 50 miles. Waters falling or flowing into this basin have no exit to the seas, except by evaporation, wind, or the bellies of animals. So we were situated neither east nor west, as it were, until we came out of the basin west of Red Desert.

Then There Is No Mountain

As we passed through Rock Springs, we crossed an old path of mine, so I told Joe and Louise about the time, in 1976, when I was 24, I'd fled Wyoming with another man's woman.

The Summer of Cherries and Trout

She and I had escaped on an eastbound train, which, in turn, led to my long Summer of Cherries and Trout. I had wanted to see the West, so, a few weeks before our escape back east, I'd saved up a little money, quit my dead-end job at the end of a dreary Indiana winter, and caught a train to Denver.

At Denver, I changed to a different train, an old fashioned train with wood and brass trim, heavy silverware, and linen napkins in the dining car. It chugged up into the mountains, and over the Great Divide, and then out through the desert to Salt Lake City. From Salt Lake City, I hitchhiked over to Jackson Hole, Wyoming, to look for work at one of the ski resorts. It hadn't snowed there all winter. No one had come to ski. The shopkeepers had grown surly by the time I got there, in early March. There were no in-town jobs, but I found a job with a survey crew, working up in the mountains, mapping the layers of strata below the surface. We worked in the Salt River Range around Afton. We'd ride in the crew trucks for an hour or so in the mornings to a couple of helicopters, then take the helicopters up into the mountains and go to work. We laid out a line of geophones, which functioned essentially like old-fashioned telephone mouthpieces, and wired them together and back to a booth with a seismographic pin reader. Then we laid a parallel line of low-power explosives at regular intervals. When we set off the explosives, the line of geophones picked up the echoes from the strata below and fed them as electrical impulses to the pin reader in the hut, which graphed the results.

In the evenings, we'd make the run back to the saloons, cafes, and hotels of Afton, Smoot, or Alpine, depending on where we were working. We kept up a running poker game that moved from room to room, and town to town. Our crew was made up of a couple dozen young adventurers from all over, male and female, couples and singles.

A contingent of our crew declined the hotels and stayed in a tent and teepee camp located outside of whatever town we were working from. They were different from the rest of us. They wore leather and feathers. They were, men and women alike, lean and sun-cured. When their eyes weren't looking right at you, they seemed to be looking somewhere else altogether. While we were based out of Alpine, a certain green-eyed woman from the camp group and I became attracted to each other. But she'd come there with her man. They'd been backpacking for a couple of years in Central America and the North American West.

We arranged a couple of secret liaisons before we got caught. Neither of us bothered with lies about love. We had a few stolen minutes in my room where we tugged at each other's clothes, and pressed our flesh together. Soon after our second rendezvous, I opened my door to answer an insistent knock, and it was her man. I should have known that our meetings wouldn't be secret for long. Standing in my doorway, wearing a look of wounded pride, he confronted me, his fingers gripping and ungripping at his sides. He struggled to keep his fingers from reaching for my throat, or forming a fist and punching me in the jaw. His voice was strained, and his words choked-off. I got the message, though. I'd stolen from him, and humiliated him, and we were going to have trouble if I stuck around. After making sure I'd gotten the message, he turned and stomped down the hall. I locked the door and packed my bags, proving myself a coward as well as a thief.

There was a bridge over the Snake River right outside Alpine. I gave a note to the green-eyed woman's best friend to deliver to her explaining that I was going to camp under that bridge for the night, and then I would hitch-hike down to Rock Springs, a couple hundred miles south, where I would wait for her if she cared to come. I told her I'd go to the train station every day at 8 a.m. and 4 p.m. to look for her. And so I did. At Rock Springs I found an old hotel near the station. Not wanting to pay for a room, I climbed up the fire escape to the roof where I rolled out my sleeping bag and slept under the stars each night for three nights, among the scattered remains of previous camps. On the third morning, as I came around to the front of the hotel on my way to the station, she came out of the hotel lobby. I could have slept in her bed if I'd known.

We caught a train east to Des Moines and hitchhiked north to Minneapolis, where she knew people. When we arrived in Minneapolis, it was late May, and the city sparkled happily under crisp clean blue northern skies. Her friends, a young married couple, had a downtown apartment. They welcomed her with hugs and highly amused smiles. Since they'd last seen her, she'd backpacked over much of the Western Hemisphere, and now here she was at their door, her skin burnished by faraway suns and winds, her green eyes seeming paler, on the run from love, boy toy in tow. We struggled out of our backpacks in their foyer and set up camp on the floor of their spare bedroom, which had no bed. They seemed to be glad for the disruption we caused in their routine, although they were also friends, or at least acquaintances, with her man. They worked during the day and we all made meals together in the evenings, and we kept the conversations light.

Everyone understood that our situation was temporary, but no one knew just how it would end. Their apartment had hardwood floors, and big old windows that actually worked, through which bright colorful slabs of light poured onto the floor, and across their oval rug, in the afternoons. After we'd been there a little over a week, I happened to be sitting alone in their apartment watching their cat slowly chase the moving pool of light, and listening to the radio (classic rock before it acquired "classic" status), when the phone rang. I'd begun to feel at home enough to answer their phone.

"Hello," I said.

"Hello. Who's this?"

"Richard."

There was a moment of silence. "Well, this is—-." It was the green-eyed woman's man. He'd found us.

"Oh. Where are you?"

"I'm at the airport. I need a ride to the apartment."

There was another moment of silence. "I'll tell them." I hung up, and started packing.

By the time she and the woman with whom we were staying came through the door a few minutes later, bearing groceries, I was packed. I told her that her man was at the airport and needed a ride to the apartment, and that I needed a ride to the train station. Her green eyes didn't even blink. At the station she bought me a ticket to South Bend, Indiana. Then, she kissed me quickly on the cheek and left for the airport. I was headed to South Bend because she had a friend whose family had a cherry orchard just north of Traverse City, Michigan.

She said the cherries were ripening soon, and that they always needed hands for the harvest. She said she'd call ahead, so they'd be expecting me. She said they had migrant shacks and I could stay in one. Once I was off the train I hitchhiked north to Traverse City, and began my long Summer of Cherries and Trout. Everything she said turned out true.

The orchard was about ten miles out on the peninsula that separates Grand Traverse Bay into two halves. I introduced myself to the family standing in their front yard. The farmer and I shook hands, and I was hired with little more than a nod. The cherries, however, were still ripening. I was at least two weeks too early. My recent lover's friend was the farmer's daughter. She was about my age.

She gave me a lift for the mile or so back down the road to the row of migrant shacks. None of the Mexican workers had arrived yet, so I had my pick of accommodations. My room was a cinderblock cell in a row of like cells. I had a south-facing window, a bare electric light bulb centered in the ceiling, a one-burner hotplate, a dorm-size refrigerator, a Formica table with two chairs, and a very squeaky single bed. There was an outdoor shower, and an old wringer-style washing machine, also outside, under a porch roof tacked to the back of the building. A row of outhouses stood off by itself. The migrant camp was set among miles of orchards—cherries, plums, prunes, apples, and peaches, planted over rolling dunes. I unfurled my sleeping bag on the bed, and set my few things out on the table.

The farmer's daughter gave me a ride into Traverse City, where I spent most of my meager funds on groceries, and a cheap coffee percolator. Along the way we chatted about our mutual friend, and told each other about ourselves. All the while, we were looking each other over. She was going to be around for a couple of weeks before returning to the east coast, where she'd been living.

She came to visit me alone a few times before she left, and before the Mexicans arrived. A very squeaky bed, indeed. A few times, we went into Traverse City with friends of hers, particularly a young couple who lived in a stone cottage on the wooded shore of Bowers Harbor. They had a beehive, and a garden. Dried herbs hung from their front porch roof. He had a beard, and she had hairy legs. Their yellow dog wore a red bandanna. They were always overflowing with laughter. The four of us would go out to a hoppin' jukejoint called The Sawmill *(motto: You'll never get bored feet at The Sawmill!)* to eat cheeseburgers, drink beer, and listen to rowdy stringbands stomp it out for the dancers.

I ran out of money before the cherries got ripe. I'd been boiling eggs in a Campbell's soup can, and to supplement my egg diet I roamed the orchards looking for early cherries but there wasn't much to be had, although I found nice stands of wild asparagus. When I wasn't foraging, I sometimes sat outside my door in the sun, leafing through "The Whole Earth Catalogue," or studying "The Dome Builder's Handbook," planning my dream home. I was getting hungry when I heard about a strawberry farm in a town on the west bank of the bay, where the strawberries were ripe and needed picking. I made my way over there and they hired me on the spot. Picking strawberries is some of the hardest work I've ever done. Pure stoop labor. My back hurt continually while I worked there. I worked and slept among large families of Mexicans. They tended to have nice pickups, and lots of kids, and everyone worked. They all, from the oldest to the youngest, could beat me to the end of the row, every time. I seemed to be the only English-speaker in the fields, a young gringo, and so a curiosity among them. Every day I made just enough money to pay for my supper that night. I wasn't getting ahead, but I was getting by. I ate a lot of strawberries–so many that by the time I'd left, I'd developed a slightly allergic reaction to them. I'd also lost my taste for them. It would be years before I could stand the smell of strawberries again.

The migrant quarters on the strawberry farm, where I slept, I remember as a large outbuilding with a warren of tacked-together cubicles that served as bedrooms. When I lay in bed I could hear voices speaking in Spanish from the cubicles around me. The cubicle next to mine was occupied by a very young married couple. I listened to them lying in bed together, talking low, and laughing quietly. I could tell they were lying very close together. Understanding the words would only have distracted me from the sweet music of *amor* in their voices. I don't know that I've ever heard a more beautiful sound since.

In working the Michigan fruit harvest, I was following in my parents' footsteps. When they were newlyweds, they traveled north from the Ozarks with some friends to Benton Harbor, Michigan, to pick fruit. I have a snapshot of them taken that summer. They are very young. She's sixteen, he's twenty one. He has his arm around her shoulder. He has a cigarette dangling from the other hand. He's wearing a t-shirt and jeans. His hair is James Dean style, but it's 1947, well before James Dean. She's leaning into his shoulder. Her arms are crossed. She's wearing white, loose slacks, a white blouse, and a white scarf around her black hair, tied in the front. They are both looking right into the camera, but they don't seem to be looking into a camera. Their faces are relaxed and friendly-looking. Their un-self-conscious expressions are like those of someone who's listening to you, rather than someone posing for a picture.

When we'd finished the strawberry crop, I hitchhiked back over to my shack on the peninsula, but the cherries still weren't quite ready, and I was as broke as before. My farmer's daughter was gone but my hairy friends with the cottage fed me a couple of meals, and then gave me a fishing pole and a small tackle box. In my rambles through the orchards, I'd found a farm a half-mile or so to my west with a couple of ponds out back of the house, just beyond the barn. At dusk, I walked through the orchard, climbed a fence, crossed a lush hay meadow, climbed another fence, and slipped up to the pond and went fishing. I fished mostly by feel, as I kept my eyes on the house, which was lit up for the evening. Among the yellow lights, I could see the blue glow of the TV flickering, so I felt pretty safe.

The pond was stocked with trout. Overstocked, in my opinion. They were so hungry, I got a bite on every cast. They especially liked the red and yellow Rooster Tail I was tossing at them. Within ten minutes I had three good, pan-sized trout on my stringer. I was so hungry I could hardly wait to eat them. When I climbed the fence to the hay meadow, my figure atop the fence spooked a couple of horses loitering there in the low evening light. Back at the shack I rigged up a grill and built a fire of apple deadwood in the yard. While it was burning down, I gutted the fish, and when the fire was right, I grilled them. I can still taste them. Every fish I've eaten since has been and still is measured against that meal. After I'd eaten, I perked up a cup of coffee and drank it and looked into the fire. After that I played the harmonica for a while. I played the only song I knew: "I'm So Lonesome I Could Cry". I played it over and over, putting different kinds of English on it, until the fire died out.

The cherries finally got ripe, the harvest got under way, and I had money in my pocket and groceries in my shack. I also had company in the camp. A large Mexican-American family had arrived in their late-model bright red Ford pickup with a white camper shell. They spoke English, so we got acquainted a little. They worked an annual circuit from Brownsville, Texas, up through the Midwest for tomatoes, and to Michigan for summer fruits, then over to upstate New York for apples, and then down to Florida for oranges and grapefruits, and then back over to Brownsville to rest before starting out again. Brownsville was home for them.

I got along really well with their kids, three or four little boys with big mischievous grins, and a couple of giggling little girls, all running and rolling around the yard. The boys called me Beatle, because of my long hair. I asked the boys to teach me Spanish. They enthusiastically agreed to teach Beatle Spanish. "How do you say 'car'?" I asked them. I was sitting in my chair outside my door. They were gathered around me. *"Carro!"* they all yelled over each other. "Carro," I repeated back. *"Si!"* they shouted. "How do you say 'girl'?" *"Chica!"* "Chica?" *"Si! Yes!"* My lessons went well for a few minutes, but then I began to suspect that they were pulling my leg because every word I asked them about, they just added "o" and shouted it back at me, collapsing into each other with laughter. "How do you say 'cherry'?" *"Cherrio!"* "How do you say 'coffee'?" *"Coffee-o!"* "Really?" *"Really-o!"* "I think you boys are pulling my leg!" *"Leg-o!"* I chased them away. They scattered, hollering "Beatle-o" over their shoulders. From then until the day they pulled out, I was Beatle-o.

On my evening fishing trips, I became acquainted with the two horses in the hay meadow. The spot where I crossed the fence was at an apple tree. The horses had eaten all the green apples they could reach. One evening I picked a couple of apples which I held out to them. They came up to me and each took an apple. They seemed to go delirious with happiness, chomping away, shaking their heads and slinging great long strings of foamy saliva around, getting some on me. After that, whenever they saw me coming, they galloped across the meadow to meet me, already foaming at the mouth, and I stopped to feed them apples. One night I caught an especially large trout. He was 22 inches long and bigger around than my arm. He put up a heck of a fight, dancing on top of the water, leaping and diving. It took a while to get him to shore. His splashes were so loud I was afraid the family, or the family dog, might hear the commotion. While I was reeling him in, I felt like I was racing against the moment when the backyard light would come on, and the dog would come charging my way. Once I got the fish on the bank, I strung him and hightailed it back to the shack. It took me three days to finish eating that fish.

After the cherries came the plums, and after the plums the prunes, and after the prunes the peaches, and after the peaches the apples. Between each ripening was a lull, so my fortunes rose and fell over the summer. During the harvests I stocked up on groceries, and during the lulls, I gleaned for leftover fruits that had escaped being harvested, and visited my farm pond almost nightly. Now and then my friends from the cottage would pick me up and take me to town to shop and go to The Sawmill. I was doing okay.

After the peach harvest, I decided to move on. It was going to be a good long while before the apples were ready. I found a job in southern

Michigan working on a survey crew for a couple of weeks. Once I got my first paycheck, I hitchhiked home to Richmond, Indiana, a couple hundred miles south.

When I stepped into my parents' house, outside Richmond, I was just in time for supper. Everyone was there—Mom, Dad, brothers and sister, girlfriends, wives, husband, kids, and pets. It was awfully nice to be back in the fold. It had just turned September. They told me I'd lost a lot of weight since they'd seen me in March. I guess cherries and trout is a pretty low-fat diet.

Green River to Twin Falls–No Wifi!

As Joe, Louise and I passed by the town of Green River, Wyoming, Joe told us about one-armed John Wesley Powell's thrilling 1869 expedition down the unexplored Green and Colorado Rivers in wooden boats. Louise, sitting in the back, had withdrawn into herself.

After Evanston we rode a long, beautiful descent into Utah to the interchange of I-80 and I-84, which is an impressive feat of highway engineering with an improbably small footprint in a tight canyon. We exited I-80 onto I-84. We cut across Utah alongside backwaters from Great Salt Lake, past Ogden, where they drove the Golden Spike to complete the first coast-to-coast railway way back when, and Brigham City with the Wasatch Range in the background, and Logan. You know you've been in Wyoming when Utah seems overpopulated.

Once we cleared the I-15 split at Trementon, the land emptied of people and roads, and in the hour of dusk we saw two horses, one with an empty saddle, walking in single file through the sagebrush from one unknowable place to another. In a few moments the scene was well behind us but it had caused a strange feeling to come over us. Was there a cowboy lying snakebit or brokelegged in some hidden fold? There didn't seem to be a scenario to explain what we'd seen wherein the cowboy would come out okay. The image of that riderless horse added a layer of anxiety to the blackness rising around us. "There was a time," Joe ventured, "when, if we saw something like that, we'd stop whatever we were doing and go looking for the man. There was a time when you just wouldn't have felt like you had a choice."

I nodded, and said, "Yup." But I was thinking that these were still those times for anybody who might be out there themselves and came across those horses. But we weren't out there, were we? And we couldn't be blamed, could we, if we didn't even take the Land Rover cruise control off of 85 as those horses and their unsettling mystery diminished and disappeared in our rear view mirrors. They'd vanished within seconds. On the Interstate, we felt as separated from the land we passed through as from the imaginary world of a movie screen. The only thing imaginary, though, was our feeling of separation. One false move could put us out there with that cowboy. It was something to think about as the closing credits of the last day of Spring rolled slowly down, and finally faded to a profound, desolate, new-moon black. We sailed northwest onto the Snake River Plain.

When Twin Falls lit up the horizon like a mini-Vegas we were all glad to call it a day, road-weary after a thirteen-hour drive. Louise had been withdrawn all day, refusing to be pulled in to our desultory conversations, and when I'd quietly asked her a couple of times if she was okay, she'd just replied with a brittle "I'm fine!" and looked away. After checking into a Motel 6, we had a little pillow talk before falling asleep. I learned that she was sulking over our last night in Boulder, and my admission that night that I hadn't cared one way or the other whether she'd wanted to go to the bookstore with Joe and me. She hadn't wanted to go, but she'd wanted me to want her to go, or something like that. I was too sleepy to even be confused, and we both were soon fast asleep.

I woke up early and went for a run, after which I stopped by the motel lobby, poured a cup of complimentary coffee, and took it to Louise. She was just waking up. I saw Joe outside the room, and we agreed to walk down the street for breakfast. Louise asked that we bring her back something. She wanted to shower and primp a bit. Over breakfast and coffee at some chain place, Joe said that he wanted to find a place with wi-fi and better coffee. We had a long way to go to get to Portland. I cringed at the thought of waiting around while Joe sipped coffee and browsed the internet. Our hosts in Portland–our old friends, Nicole and Lisa—were planning to prepare supper for us. And Louise and I had been keenly anticipating visiting Shoshone Falls. This site on the Snake River, and the tourists it draws, is the main reason for Twin Falls' continuing existence.

"Well, Joe, we've got a lot to do today," I said. "We really want to show you Shoshone Falls, and Louise wants to do a watercolor of it. "It's early yet," he replied, unmoved. Our conversation then drifted back to where it always did in those days—sharing the growing excitement of our impending climb of Mt. Rainier. We'd be checking into the Whittaker Bunkhouse at Rainier Base Camp in less than 36 hours, if all went according to plan. After breakfast and two cups of coffee, we checked out and delivered Louise's breakfast back at the Motel 6. We loaded the Land Rover while she ate. When she'd finished, we climbed aboard. Louise and I hadn't spoken much, but her mood was much improved. She, like me, was eager to visit Shoshone Falls, and cheered by the prospect. I looked at my watch and the map. "Shall we head over to the Falls?" I suggested to Joe. "I need some wi-fi first," he replied.

"My God, this place is ugly!" Joe exclaimed as we drove up and down the streets of Twin Falls looking for a place with free wi-fi, and he was right. "There's nothing here more than twenty years old at the most," he added, again rightly, as we looked over the crass concentration of franchises, chain stores, and motels, all of whose names you know. If there is an old section of Twin Falls, Idaho, it has been obscured by rampant development, rendering the place an example of banal American anonymity. Twin Falls is identical to a thousand beltway developments at the edges of cities all over the country—except that in Twin Falls there is no beltway, and no actual city that we could locate. Los Angeles has been famously described as a thousand suburbs in search of a city. Twin Falls is one suburb in search of a city.

"Well, at least it hasn't devolved into self-parody," I said, which was the faintest of praise. I was thinking of places like Branson, Dodge City, Gatlinburg, Williamsburg, Las Vegas, and others. "At least there isn't a faux-Old West street with shootouts on the hour, and blacksmiths making useless horseshoes."

Joe said, "That's true. No one's pretending here. What you see is what you get. What I want is some wi-fi." We pulled in to a McDonald's. Louise and I waited in the Rover while Joe checked. He came back outside scowling. "They want to charge for wi-fi!" he reported. "What the hell?" We rolled down the street, searching the signage for possible wi-fi connections. "There's a Starbucks!" We made one of our U-turns, accompanied by a now-familiar honking of horns from other drivers, and pulled in. Joe emerged five minutes later, and climbed aboard. "Bastards. I am *not* paying for wi-fi." It was mid-morning by now.

"Want to give it up?" I asked hopefully, but Joe seemed to have an idée-fixe of himself relaxing in a public venue sipping coffee and gazing into his laptop, partaking of free wi-fi, and he was determined to make it so.

"There's got to be a place!" he insisted. We drove around some more. "Hah! Barnes and Noble!" We all went inside. I visited the restroom and when I came out Joe was storming out the door. Louise looked at me with an unreadable expression.

Back in the Rover, Joe said, "I can't believe these sons of bitches! Well, I guess we should just go, head out, get on the way to Portland. We've wasted enough time in this dump." Suddenly, he was in a hurry.

"No, Joe! Louise and I have been looking forward to going to Shoshone Falls for *months*. Louise wants to make a painting there. *We want to go to the falls.*"

A Visit to Shoshone Falls

"Well, how the hell far is it?"

"Two or three miles. Come on, let's just go."

Reluctantly, Joe pulled out in the direction of the falls. "How long is it going to take you to make your painting?" he asked Louise churlishly. I looked back at her. She had tears of anger in her eyes. She said nothing, nor did I. It was an unanswerable question.

At Shoshone Falls, Louise and I walked together and Joe walked alone. She was bitterly angry at Joe. There was zero chance that she was going to set up and paint. The necessary frame of mind had been crushed by his insensitivity. When I tried to empathize with her, she told me she was just as angry at me for not standing up for her. "But I *did* stand up for you!" I defended myself. "Look, we're here! You can paint if you choose! Look around, feel the spray, hear the thunder. What more could I have done?"

"You could have beat him up for me."

"What? Louise, I'm 57 years old. I don't beat people up, and even if I did, I don't think I could beat Joe up, even if I wanted to, which I don't." She rolled her eyes, and sighed at the idiot male who was always taking her literally when he shouldn't (the present moment, for example) and never taking her literally when he should (most other moments). "He knows Hopkido, you know!" I added.

She walked to the overlook, leaving both me and her anger behind. I followed her. At the overlook we became soaked by blowing mist from the falls below us. The Snake River drains the Tetons over in Wyoming and carries all that water down onto the Snake River Plain, where it has cut a narrow chasm through the basalt that underlies the patchy topsoil and runs across much of southern Idaho. Down in that crack, Shoshone Falls—once described as "The Niagara of the West"—takes the chasm a couple of hundred feet deeper, in thunder and mist. Beneath the chasm, they say the fires of Hell come pretty close to the surface, in the form of a tectonic "hot spot." They say that a series of "supervolcanoes" effectively bulldozed a swath through the Rocky Mountains, obliterating them and creating the Snake River plain. You can see this on any large scale topographic map of the American West.

We speculated about where Thomas Moran had set up his easel, although we'd never see the falls as he'd seen them in 1900, when he immortalized them in an enormous painting. That painting is on permanent display at the Gilcrease Museum in Tulsa.

The developers had been busy down there, marring the view with an assemblage of McMansions perched just above the falls and a power station at its base stringing electric lines across the chasm. There are two kinds of people in the world, in situations like this: those who look beyond the beauty to find the ugly, and those who look beyond the ugly to find the beauty. Which kind, I asked myself, did I want to be?

We were there on a sunny morning, which created a bright vivid rainbow in the consoling mists blowing up around us. In a few minutes, bad feelings bathed away, we took photos of the rainbow, bought a tee-shirt at the little booth nearby, and rejoined Joe, who had sprinted up to the top and back down along the access road. On the way out we stopped at a stand of sagebrush and I cut off a branch to take back home to Tulsa. It saturated the Rover with such an overpowering aroma that we tied it off inside a plastic garbage bag. It still permeated the Rover, but at an acceptable level.

As we pulled past the last Bed, Bath & Beyond, and beyond, it occurred to me that things hadn't gone that well in Twin Falls.

Twin Falls to Portland

We followed the Snake out of Idaho on I-84. West of Boise, agriculture peters out to treeless sagebrush hills, which grow wilder and wilder as you draw closer to Oregon. Louise and Joe seemed to have forgotten about Shoshone Falls. They chatted amiably about art (her passion) and history (his passion) and art history (common ground). Most everything I know about these subjects, I've learned from one of them or the other. Still, lacking their formal educations, I tend to be left with the present when the subject turns to history—which is fine with me really—although in that particular present, I was peering out the windows, looking for a vestige of history. We were following the old Oregon Trail, and I was looking for its trace on the hillsides as we crossed the river into Oregon at the town of Ontario. Having seen and walked the old Santa Fe Trail in Oklahoma, I knew what to look for. Somewhere just past Farewell Bend, where the Trail parts ways with the river, my vigilance was rewarded as I spotted the old trace arcing up over a hill on our left. Then we plunged further into the loneliness of Eastern Oregon.

I've never been anywhere else as lonely-seeming as that country. The dreadful, ominous beauty of those endless layers of dry sagebrush-and-grass folds fading to an unreachable horizon under the cobalt sky diminished us to our true insignificance. We were a microscopic black dot barely moving at 75mph along a slender dotted line.

After a brief rest and fuel stop in Baker City, we passed La Grande and headed up the Blue Mountains and over Deadman Pass. I was driving, and as we cleared the pass, I shared with Joe and Louise a vivid memory of taking this westbound pass a few years before when I was an over-the-road trucker. The western descent is steep and long, and the view ahead and below makes you feel like you're looking down from an airplane. "I'd not had much experience at the time, and I hadn't enough sense to use my Jake Brake," I said. "So, I was trying to check my speed with just gears and air brakes, which was a big mistake on a grade this steep. I had eighty-thousand pounds pushing me down the hill. So, when I got to about here, where we are right now, I looked in my mirrors and saw hot blue smoke coming out from my trailer wheels. If they got too hot and failed, I'd be in a world of hurt. I mean just look out there." Joe was doing everything he could to *avoid* looking out there as we rounded the curves.

"Well, I had to pull over and sit there for thirty minutes 'til my brakes cooled off. After that, I kept her in a low gear and babied her on down around the bend, watching for smoke all the time, until I got to the last section, down there, which is just about a perfectly straight ramp down to the desert floor. Once I got around the last bend, I took the truck out of gear and let that trailer just push me as hard as it wanted. I was practically in flight by the time I leveled out at the bottom." We glided easily in the Rover around a hairpin curve.

"Yeah. How about slowing it down a bit?" Joe was staring into the dashboard as he made this request. He sounded calm but he spoke through clamped teeth.

"Okay. Hey, you see that emergency truck ramp up there?" I pointed to a steep upward ramp carved into the mountainside, coming off the highway. It was paved with deep gravel to its abrupt top end at a row of orange barrels.

"What about it?"

"Those things always give me an uneasy feeling. I used to speculate about them a lot when I was trucking in the mountains. I always wondered if I'd have the guts to ditch into one of them if I was coming down too fast for the roadway. I mean, in a situation like that, none of the voices hollering at you from inside want to admit that you're no longer in control of your vehicle. It's got to be a very difficult split-second decision to override them, admit that you've lost it, and intentionally take your truck off the pavement and onto the ramp. I've always feared that I'd fly right on past it, unable to make that decision, until it was about ten feet too late. In a situation like that, *any* too late is way too late."

"Yeah. Mm hmm. You're gonna slow it down, now, right?"

We stopped in Pendleton for a Starbucks and a stretch. Joe took the wheel. We pulled out onto the street, made our customary wrong turn/U-turn combination, got back onto the highway and headed west. A little past Hermiston we came abreast of the Columbia River. So strange to see such a broad, muscular river flowing through such arid land. We followed along her bank all the rest of the way to Portland. Somewhere between Hermiston and The Dalles, we saw Mount Hood shining white, towering above everything else. Just past the place where Hood River empties into the Columbia, everything changes in a short space from sere desert to lush temperate rainforest. The solstice sun had slipped down low when we finally rounded a bend and found ourselves face to face with Portland's brightly lit skyline, and its reflection in the Willamette River.

Nicole and Lisa

I got us into Nicole and Lisa's part of town, working from memory, but hailing from the cities of the plains, with their simple grid layouts, we inevitably got lost in Portland's spaghetti-bowl streets. We pulled over and called our hosts. Lisa assured us we weren't far and gave us directions. We circled their neighborhood for several minutes, unable to pin her directions onto the writhing streets. A half-dozen U-turns later we gave up and called again, got a refined set of directions, and finally found their street, their block, and their house, with Lisa standing outside cheerfully waving us in.

It was wonderful to see Nicole and Lisa again. Louise was especially happy to be released from her confinement with two troublesome males, and in their friendly female embraces again. They welcomed us all with open arms and ushered us into their dining room, where one of Louise's paintings was hung on the wall. "You men are going to climb a mountain! You need meat!" they declared. The table was set, and in the center was a platter piled high with aromatic, thinly sliced marinated flank steak, hot from the pan, surrounded by various delectable looking side dishes, and accompanied by a bottle of Willamette Valley red wine. Their windows were open and the air was fresh. Soon the road and all its stresses dissolved away from us as we ate, drank, laughed, and talked with ever-loosening tongues about the road, about Rainier, about Nicole and Lisa's lives, and everything under the sun.

When the meal broke up, the evening sky still held light so we decided to have a walk. Lisa and Louise went one way, because they both like to dawdle along, while Nicole led Joe and me in another way, to their neighborhood park. Nicole is light and quick. Quick of mind, quick of tongue, and, we soon discovered, quick of foot. We followed her up and down the neighborhood hills at a walk that was just this side of a run. She talked over her shoulder the whole time. The way through the park included a path through a short section of deep, dark, old-growth evergreen woods. As soon as I entered that shadowy place, I tuned out the ongoing conversation between Nicole and

Joe, and slowed to a near stop. I lagged behind, padding silently under the big trees, among the ferns and vines, following the path along a tiny murmuring stream. Unfamiliar birds flitted around in my peripheral vision up among the dark branches. I could hear others singing last lullabies, hidden in the bushes. Frogs and crickets had added their songs. Heady smells of night had begun to rise. Nicole and Joe stopped up ahead and looked back at me. "You're missing this!" I called out. They paid me no mind, talking away, getting to know each other, while I strolled up to them. We then continued our fast pace out of the shadows, across the park, past its community garden, and back to Nicole's street and home, all three of us talking nonstop the whole way. We arrived home feeling flushed and energized.

Their home is roomy and airy, with good flow. Three stories rise over a steeply sloping lot, with a generous, two-level deck providing a deep view of the hills of west Portland. Louise and Lisa eventually came home from their stroll and we all sat in the living room visiting, taking turns stroking their two cats and their sweet old dog, until we got sleepy. I went to off to the same bed that Louise and I had slept in on our last visit, and before too long Louise joined me. We lay close together in the dark and whispered drowsily for a few minutes, before falling asleep.

Next morning, we all stood around in the kitchen chatting over coffee as Nicole and Lisa danced around each other with practiced ease, preparing a breakfast fit for Paul Bunyan. Their kitchen is presided over by an old black and white photo of a young Julia Child towering over a tiny, humble stove in her kitchen in France. The stove seemed to come up only to her waist as she stood there in a dress, apron, and high heels with a skillet in her hand, smiling at the camera.

Nicole, who had just published a cookbook, "Baking Unplugged," told us that this photo was a big part of the inspiration for her book. "People these days like to say that they can't bake, because they don't have all the high-tech modern gadgetry they need and blah, blah, blah. Well, just look at Julia there. Neither did she! That's no reason not to bake. People have been baking for thousands of years without a Viking commercial oven or whatever. So, I created some recipes and directions for how to make them with just simple low-tech kitchen tools and equipment. Baking unplugged."

Louise would be staying with our friends in Portland while Joe and I climbed Rainier. After our huge breakfast, Joe and I futzed with our gear for a while, and reloaded it all into the Land Rover just so, minus Louise's luggage. We all gathered outside, where Joe and I were each hugged briefly and wished luck by each of the women. I saved Louise for last and we held each other close for a few seconds and whispered to each other. Then Joe held up his ice axe, and instructed me to do the same, for what he said was a mountaineering tradition. He then told Louise, Lisa, and Nicole to each grasp our axe handles for a moment, so that we could take a part of them, in spirit, up to the summit. Lisa handed us a bag with sandwiches made from home-baked baguettes stuffed with the previous night's steak leftovers. We pulled out of the driveway feeling grand, turned left, went half a block, realized we should have turned right, made a corrective U-turn, and drove back past them, waving and smiling down the hill.

On to Rainier!

We took I-5 north to U.S. 12 east, and then State Highway 7 north to Elbe, then east again on 706 to Ashford. I don't remember just where we were when we first saw Mount Rainier, but I remember how her white cone pierced the blue sky and how she dwarfed the green lowlands gathered around her wide skirts. She slipped in and out of view as we undulated through lush rural Washington, emerging clearer and bigger every time she showed herself again. *"First there is a mountain, then there is no mountain, then there is,"* we sang.

At Ashford, we pulled into Rainier Base Camp, elevation 1,764 feet, which was operated by our guide service, Rainier Mountaineering Incorporated. RMI has a long history on Rainier, and a close association with Whittaker Mountaineering. We checked into the Whittaker Bunkhouse, a nicely old-fashioned wood-frame building with a wraparound porch lined by small, Spartan rooms with wooden floors and wood-frame windows. That afternoon we met up with our guides and the other sixteen climbers who'd gathered for our group climb. "Let's just all introduce ourselves," our guides recommended, once they'd taken a roll call. "Tell everyone your name, where you're from, and why you want to climb Mount Rainier."

Why?

Joe and I had each been asked this question often during our eight months of training and preparation in Tulsa, and at first we felt challenged to come up with reasons more substantial than mere curiosity. We'd sigh, affect faraway looks, and mumble in half sentences about man's need to explore, to go where the crowd can't, and about the purity of high places. Then we'd look into our questioner's eyes, and explain that a mountain is something to measure yourself against. Something to measure your *fitness* against, fitness being a word with connotations beyond the physical. In our self-consciousness, we might have put on a show of irony, but, really, we meant every word of it.

Then There Is No Mountain

But what about mere curiosity? Shouldn't it have been enough to say that we were just curious about how the air feels up there? What shade of blue the sky? How far you can see? My own reasons for climbing Mount Rainier were all of the above, but I didn't tell them that when my turn came.

A State of Grace

Here's something else I didn't tell them: One day in early spring, 2008, when Joe's pestering me about climbing mountains had begun to die down, I was told by a doctor that I had prostate cancer. The news was not completely unexpected. Despite three excruciating biopsies that had each turned out negative, blood tests and an enlarged prostate gland had been suggesting, more and more insistently, that I had cancer. I'd lost twenty pounds, for no apparent reason, in about three months. I've always had a stable metabolism. In thirty years, my weight hasn't varied more than five pounds, no matter how much I eat or don't eat, no matter how much I exercise or don't. When I'd visited my brother Mike earlier that spring, whom I hadn't seen in six months, he was alarmed at my weight loss. I'd been working out regularly at a gym and had never felt better. I told him and others that I'd just shed fat, and that my weight loss was a side-effect of fitness. I really believed it, since three biopsies had found nothing.

When I was told that the fourth biopsy tested positive for cancer, I felt as if someone had knocked me off my feet with a hard blow to my chest. The news came over the phone, while I was at work. A nurse said, with a callous matter-of-factness that I later came to admire: "Mr. Higgs, we got the results from your biopsy, and it is positive. You do have prostate cancer. The doctor would like to see you as soon as possible to review your options. We suggest that you bring your wife along with you." I went straight home, and told Louise, who cried out and collapsed in tears onto the sofa. We spent the afternoon comforting each other. We met the doctor next morning. There were three options: surgery, radiation, nothing. The doctor advised me to take a little time, not too much, and make a decision. Within a few days, I picked myself up, dusted myself off and got busy. After researching the question, mostly online, I decided surgery was best for me. A date was set for three months ahead—early August.

Then There Is No Mountain

I prepared for surgery like a fighter preparing for a fight, concentrating on physical and mental discipline. I worked out hard in the gym four times a week, and took yoga lessons twice a week. Louise prepared us meals from fresh, wholesome foods. My friend Anitra recommended that I read Eckhardt Tolle's "A New Earth." Joe gave me his well-thumbed copy of Shunryu Suzuki's "Zen Mind, Beginner's Mind." I read them both daily. These books changed my life.

The routines of work and chores usually kept me preoccupied. I didn't dwell on my cancer consciously, but there were several episodes when paralyzing anxiety attacks would well up to the surface without warning. And without regard to where I was or what I was doing or who I was with.

One June morning, after such an episode the night before, I called in sick, packed a couple of sandwiches and some water, and left Louise a note. I drove an hour and a half northwest of Tulsa to the Tallgrass Prairie Preserve, up in the Osage Nation. The preserve is 40,000 acres of open, rolling grasslands and freeform patches of crosstimber oak forests. I pulled off a gravel road out in the big middle of it, got out of the pickup and started walking. By the time my pickup had diminished to a blue dot, I'd become nicely winded, and I'd slipped into a state of grace.

With every inhale, I pulled in everything—the high, thin clouds scrawled across the sky, the bright patches of white flowers near and far jittering hypnotically in the wind, the countless singing birds jumping like grasshoppers out of the waist-high grass in a rolling wave before me, the spicy pollens that landed on my tongue and also smudged my pant legs, and the heady smell of damp earth rising from braided streamlets coursing down through the roots and stones. With every exhale, I lost more of my Self. Breathing the world in, breathing the self out, I became diluted to the point of nonexistence.

Aware of everything yet focused on nothing, I glided weightlessly through the flowers and grasses. I seemed to hear everything with new clarity. The wind's rough whisper, bird and insect songs, swish of grass, trickle of water, all distinct, yet blended into one. I became separated from my feet, which made their own decisions and were never wrong and never stumbled. I came to rest on a shelf of stone at the top of a bluff, which placed me at a level just below the tops of the trees that had grown up along the bluff from below. I had a close-up view of the busy birdlife going on within those shaded upper branches, but I was so still, the birds took no notice of me. I may have been invisible. Down below, Sand Creek made a shiny U-turn against the bluff, bordered by redbuds still in late bloom. Rising again, taut as a sail hung from my spine, I wandered without direction, a sail without a sailor, over ridges baking in the sun, through park-like groves of postoak, and around drifting herds of bison, until I re-encountered my Self. I was back at my pickup by the side of the road. The sky was that peculiar shade of blue that I call Osage Blue, because I never see it anywhere else.

We all have moments of grace. Moments in the day that we fully in-habit, disengaged from past and future. We've all felt the transient sense of well-being that results. But such moments usually arrive unexpectedly, and they are fleeting. They fade as quickly as dreams as we're pulled back into the hurly-burly. We forget that they even transpired.

I'd never been allowed such an extended state of grace before, or, for that matter, since. I remained in its slowly loosening grip for a long time after. I suppose I still am, really, because that day is a part of me now. I call it up from time to time, and it calms me. I caution myself, however, against trying to duplicate that day, or its lesson will be lost. Bliss resides in this mo-ment only, not in memories, or wishes. That day on the prairie was a gift, and it was exactly the right gift at the right time. I know, now, what I am capable of. I had no more anxiety attacks after that.

I found that I didn't fear the cancer. I was confident we would kill it long before it had any chance to kill me. Nor did I fear the surgery. I did fear the possible after-effects of surgery, which included impotence, incontinence, and other unpleasantries best not even contemplated. I kept this fear at bay, as the date drew nearer, by focusing on my physical training, and by putting into practice what I was learning from Tolle and Suzuki. I also had long talks with Louise, who was steadfast, brave, and devoted, although I'm sure she was often struggling inside not to fall apart. When the day arrived, I was in great shape. Except for a few malevolent cancer cells multiplying deep down inside me, I'd never been healthier in my life. I was lean and tough, and ready for anything.

Family and friends gathered at the hospital on the appointed day, to see me off, it seemed. When the orderly wheeled me away from them I was calm, alert, focused and ready. Louise went with me into a small ante-room, where a nurse had me undress and make some final preparations. Then I was wheeled away from her. She didn't look too good.

The surgery they performed is known as a "robotically assisted laparoscopic prostatectomy." This amazing procedure allows them to operate with minimal blood loss and scarring, and with a degree of precision that would allow the surgeon to remove my prostate from within its sheath of nerves without damaging the nerves themselves. It would be like removing a plum from its peel without tearing the peel. Leaving those nerves intact was important. I would never have an erection again without them.

The surgeon controlled the robot by using a joystick at a computer terminal a few feet away from me. ("Just remember whose joystick you're working with, doc," I'd joked at one of our pre-surgery appointments.)

It was cold in the operating room. I remember seeing the robot. It was about nine feet tall, with six arms, and it looked like something out one of the "Terminator" movies. That's the last thing I remember. That and a quick rise of panic as they put the gas mask over my mouth and nose. It took them about two-and-a-half hours.

When I woke up, I was shivering uncontrollably, under a heavy pile of blankets. I could barely speak through my chattering teeth. An attendant told me it was normal, it was the anesthesia leaving my body, and it would subside. Some say death is cold. Being placed under general anesthesia is like rappelling face down into a cold, black abyss, and being held there suspended in that blackness. Your anesthesiologist, in the practice of his dark art, is the man holding your rope. He's the one who decides how far to lower you and when to pull you back up. When you surface into the light, you can still feel the chill.

I passed out for another while. When I woke again, the cold had gone. They wheeled me into the recovery room, where I was reunited with Louise. My prostate was missing, I had puncture wounds in my stomach and I had a catheter coming out of me. My belly had been shaved, and I was wearing nylons (for circulation, they told me). It was all pretty humiliating. I spent one night in the hospital with Louise and Joe staying by me in turns. My brother Tim, my son Robin and his girlfriend Mandy, my friend Scott, my nephew Aaron and his wife Wendy, all came by to visit during my stay. There may have been others, but I was drugged. My roommate was a highly agitated delusional alcoholic with a bad cough and a staph infection, tormented by a circling mob of demons, nurses, and germs. Joe blocked him and his swarming cloud of staph germs from getting near me, as he reeled around the room, shouting incoherently at his demons and nurses, his rolling IV stand careening in tow. I didn't get much rest, although I was sufficiently drugged that I didn't hurt. The next afternoon they released me.

I spent a dismal week strapped to a urine bag, seldom stepping outside the house, mostly just lying around reading and being taken care of by Louise, who threw her entire self into taking care of me. In the mornings, I'd have my coffee in a comfortable chair on the back patio, near my small waterfall, as the early sun warmed the back of my neck. Louise also picked up my share of our chores, which included mowing the lawn, on top of everything else. It was difficult to take without feeling guilty. After a week the catheter was removed, and after another week, the bleeding stopped. I was feeling pretty good, just sore in my gut. I had to take it easy for the next three weeks but was basically recovered. I was allowed to stay home from work for six weeks with full pay. I luxuriated in my idleness. It was the only time in my working life of 35 years that I'd been excused from working for such a period, and with no interruption in pay. I had a lot of time to think during those idle days.

What is cancer? In Medicine's ongoing argument with Death, cancer is Death's answer. For all the ways Medicine has outwitted Death to protect us from disease, Death replies: "Well, how about this, then: I'll turn your own cells against you. Your own bodies will devour themselves from within. What is your answer to that?" The answers we've stammered together so far aren't pretty, and are usually ineffectual, although they sometimes suffice. If and when Medicine comes up with a worthy response, Death will simply devise a new question, for the argument must go on.

My surgery was a complete success, with no after-effects (nerves intact!). I remain cancer-free. Looking back, in a way, I'm actually glad that it happened. It's given me gratitude. To go through your days feeling grateful is a gift in itself.

(As I write this, I'm told that 46,000,000 Americans have no health insurance. I'm not among them, thanks to a union job that includes a hard-bargained health-care package. My surgery bill was over $25,000.00. I paid $15.00. If I'd had no insurance, I'd likely be dying of cancer as I write this. If I'd had typical coverage requiring me to pay a large monthly premium, and then a large percentage of the cost of surgery, I'd likely be bankrupt as I write this. In fact, I'd likely not be writing this at all, as I'd have been financially unable to consider climbing Mt. Rainier, [even with Joe's generous underwriting of much of the cost of the trip]. For that matter, I might have been dead by now.)

One September morning, during my recovery, as I perused my shelves for something to read with my morning coffee, my fingers stopped at an old copy of Gary Snyder's translations of Han Shan's Cold Mountain poems. I hadn't opened it in years. Out on the patio, I leafed through its yellowed pages, picking and choosing poems that looked good. When I got to this one:

Clambering up the Cold Mountain Path,
The Cold Mountain trail goes on and on:
The long gorge choked with scree and boulders,
The wide creek, the mist-blurred grass.
The moss is slippery, though there's been no rain
The pine sings, but there's no wind.
Who can leap the world's ties

And sit with me among the white clouds?

—I read it once, and closed the book, remembering, with growing vividness, the night I'd first read that poem, many years before. Sad memories of troublesome times grew on themselves. Memories of the two years after high school, when I'd moved from the country to the city, pulled me deep into the past.

I Remembered The Sound of Their Laughter

I remembered the sound of their laughter, as they staggered up the steps and knocked loudly on my apartment door. When I didn't answer, they came in anyway. It was Cliff, with Marla on one arm and young Janis on the other, and a bottle of Boone's Farm apple wine gripped by the throat in each hand. "Que pasa?" Cliff said as the three of them, bumping together like loose buoys, pitched across the floor to my sofa and sprawled over it. Marla giggled. Janis closed her eyes, and a smile wafted across her face, as she settled into the cushions.

When would I learn to start locking my door? I asked myself, as I stood in the middle of my living room. "Cliff," I said. It wasn't a greeting.

I'd met Cliff soon after I'd moved to Richmond, Indiana, from the country. He'd seemed like someone who knew his way around the city—a leader to follow, and so I had. He'd seemed to me, at first, a little larger than life, because he had the ability to take over a room, but that illusion hadn't lasted very long.

"Que pasa, mi amigo? What's the haps?" He held both bottles of wine at arm's length, one stretched toward me as an offering, and one waving around out of giggling Marla's reach as she tried to snatch it from him. "Let's put some music on! It's like a tomb in here!"

"Cliff," I repeated.

"That's my name, don't—"

"Oops!" Marla cried. She'd just kicked my Chianti bottle candleholder, and my paperback of Castaneda's "A Separate Reality," off my coffee table, and onto the floor at my feet. "Really sorry, man."

"I have someone coming over," I lied, looking Cliff in the eyes. Marla captured one of the bottles.

"Is it a girl?" Cliff asked, as I returned the candleholder and book to the table and carefully set the candle back into its melted wax base.

"Yes." I lied again. I stood and watched as he took a long drink.

"That's kinda redundant, wouldn't you say?" he asked, when he came up for air. He wiped his mouth on his sleeve, and then nodded, leering, at Janis. She hadn't moved since she'd collapsed onto the sofa. Her head rested at an uncomfortable-looking angle on the sofa arm. Her hair partially covered her sixteen-year-old face. Her eyes were closed and her mouth was open. I'd seen her a couple of times at parties, and knew that she was a runaway.

Marla punched Cliff in the ribs. "Don't you dare! I'm supposed to watch out for her. Leave her alone." She glanced at me with a look that was meant to warn me to keep my hands off her young friend, but quickly lowered her eyes when she saw the anger on my face.

"What's the matter with her, anyway?" I asked Cliff, referring to Janis.

"Nothin', man. She just took a Quaalude. She's doin' fine. You want one? Make you good deal. Good deal, amigo! I can get you so messed up, you won't remember if you're datin' a girl from Eaton, or eatin' a girl from Dayton."

Marla laughed her shrill laugh and punched Cliff in the shoulder. Cliff struggled to his feet, swayed for a moment, and lurched toward my stereo. "Is she anybody we know?" he asked, referring to the someone I'd said was coming over. "Where's that new Doors record?"

"Nobody you know, Cliff. Here, I'll do that. Get back." He'd grabbed the album from the top of a stack and was jamming his blunt fingers into the cover opening trying to fish the record out.

"Well, we can't wait to meet her, Son." He surrendered the album to me and launched himself back toward the sofa.

Marla spewed wine over my coffee table as she burst into laughter at Cliff's remark. "Oops. Really sorry, man." She suppressed her laugh, and looked around for something to wipe up the wine. There was nothing in reach, so she settled back into the sofa. "Cliffy, roll us a joint, darlin'."

I put the record on. "What the hell," I said to myself, and turned it up loud. I sat down in my threadbare wingback chair by the end of the sofa nearest the stereo. The music (and an annoying, intermittent buzz in one of my speakers) would have drowned out any conversation, and there wasn't anything to say, so no one spoke as Cliff rolled a joint, lit it, and passed it to me.

"In a gadda da vida, baby," he said, with a sinister expression, as he exhaled.

When he stretched his hand to me, it exposed the scar on his wrist. I'd never asked him about the scar. The stitches spoke for themselves, and I didn't want to hear about it. With a shrug, I plucked the joint from his dirty-nailed fingers, held it up and gazed for a moment at the precious smoke curling up and away. I took a hit, and another, and another, as it came back around. By the time we'd finished the joint, the music was all that mattered.

After the Doors came Santana, then Vanilla Fudge. My neighbor, Ray, came over. He said he was tired of listening to the music through the wall. He also complained loudly that Vanilla Fudge sucked "really bad," so I replaced them with The Chambers Brothers, followed by the James Gang. Then came a friend of Ray's, who'd been looking for him, and then more people, and then some people left, and others arrived. Somehow, word had quickly spread that there was a party at my place. At some point I only knew about half the people there. Cliff remained the center of attention, keeping the party stirred up, and doing business from my sofa. Money and pills changed hands.

I had a deep aversion to taking anything I thought might be addictive (other than wine and beer), I feared mushrooms, and felt contempt for anyone who thought it was cool to give up a large portion of their paycheck for what they'd been told was cocaine, but, here in our little Midwestern city, probably wasn't. So, I stuck with pot when I felt like getting high.

I withdrew to a kitchen chair in the corner of the room, and waved away all further offerings of drink and smoke. Little John, a friend of mine from work, and an audiophile I could trust, had taken charge of the music. He touched each album only by the rim as he lifted it with his fingertips from the turntable to flip it over, or to slide it back into its paper wrapper. Before he slid the wrapper back into its cardboard cover, he turned it ninety degrees to prevent the fragile album from accidentally slipping out, and to prevent any dust from making its way into the sleeve, and onto the vinyl playing surface. Once he'd re-shelved the album, he carefully placed the next one on the turntable, lowered the needle to the groove, and lowered the turntable cover. The whole process took him about fifteen seconds. Little John was the only person I allowed to touch my turntable. In those days, there was a widespread understanding that no one touched anyone else's turntable without explicit permission—which was rarely asked, or granted.

I stepped outside for air, stood in the dark on the fractured sidewalk, and looked back at the windows of my apartment. Their puppet shadows played across my drawn shades. I was sick of them all, and sick of myself as one of them. Sick of us crowding into each others' living rooms, sick of drunken laughter, sick of amphetamine chatter, sick of hearing us ask each other where we could score. I was sick of our trying so hard to be cool.

I imagined myself walking away, walking all night, and, in the morning, renting a different apartment in a different part of town, or a different town altogether, and never going back for my stuff. I wanted to live in white, empty rooms. No furniture but a pad on the floor, bare white walls, and large, open windows. My fantasy was interrupted by a gust of wind. It blew through the old maples lining the street, and through my hair. "I wonder if Maggie's home," I asked myself, unexpectedly, and began walking toward her apartment, with the wind at my back, nudging me forward.

Maggie

"Hey, Rich. Come in." Josie, Maggie's skinny roommate, stage-whispered, swung the door open and stepped aside.

"Hey. Maggie here?" I returned her loud whisper. There were a dozen people gathered around a lanky blonde guy who was sitting in a chair strumming a guitar. I'd seen him around, but I didn't know his name. He wore a leather jacket, with fringe that swayed as he strummed.

"She's in the bedroom."

"She sleeping?"

"No."

"Oh. Is she…." I didn't want to interrupt anything. I let the question dangle.

"No, not that either," Josie giggled shyly. "I think she's reading. You can go in."

I stepped over and around people, most of whom I recognized, and pantomimed greetings, as I made my way through an invisible cloud of patchouli and pot to Maggie's bedroom door. Knocking softly, I opened it and stuck my head in. She was sitting up in bed, reading. I felt better about everything as soon as I saw her. "Hey, Maggie," I called out softly.

She smiled when she saw me and gestured me in. She set the book upside down on her patchwork quilt, to save her place. "I haven't seen you in, like, weeks. What have you been up to?"

"Oh, just working. Laying low." I sat on the bed beside her. "What are you reading?"

"Brautigan."

I reached across her and picked it up. "Revenge of the Lawn? Is it good?"

She shrugged. "It's fun. I like Brautigan."

"Me too." I reached across her again and set it back, careful to preserve her place. "So, how come you're holed up in here?"

"I couldn't take it any more."

I chuckled. "Who is the guy with the guitar?"

"He says his name is Jacques, but I didn't detect any French accent. I suspect he's from Muncie."

We laughed quietly, briefly. "So, where's what's-his-name?" I asked. I refused to say her boyfriend's name, because I hadn't approved of him.

"Larry? Gone, gone," she sighed. "And good riddance. You were right about him. How about you? You dating anybody?"

"No, not lately."

After the briefest of pauses, she changed the subject. "So, what are you reading these days, Rich?"

"Castaneda."

"Still?"

"I'm on the second book–A Separate Reality."

"I don't know about that guy, Castaneda. Some people say he's a fraud."

"You should read him for yourself. He swears every word is true. And if it is, well, my God."

We talked for a few minutes, until I suddenly had a great idea. "All right," I said, jumping up. I knew just what we needed. "Get your shoes on, Maggie, and let's go to the Dairy Queen!"

She sat upright, her glasses flashing in the lamplight. "Okay!" She clapped her hands and rubbed them together. She'd always done that, and I'd always liked it.

"I *need* a hot fudge sundae!" I said.

"Me, too!"

We emptied our pockets onto the bed, and counted our change. We had more than enough. "We'll eat like kings!" I said, as she slipped her shoes on. We passed swiftly through the gathering in the living room. Jacques was strumming away, and singing, "First there is a mountain, then there is no mountain, then there is...." A gust slammed the door behind us.

"Where's your car?" she asked.

"At home. I felt like walking. Plus, the starter's out."

A few minutes later, sitting in a booth at the Dairy Queen, I swallowed the first big bite of my sundae, and, leaning toward her, asked Maggie, in an urgent whisper, "Is there *anything* better than marijuana and hot fudge sundaes?" I looked around to make sure no one else had heard me say marijuana.

She closed her eyes as she savored her first spoonful. "Yes. One thing." she replied when she opened her eyes. "Marijuana, hot fudge sundaes and sex." She looked at me mischievously.

I just smiled. "Hot fudge sundaes are so mystical! They're cold, and yet they're hot."

"They're black, and yet they're white."

"They're liquid, and yet they're solid."

"They're chocolate, and yet they're vanilla."

"They're bitter, and yet they're sweet."

"First there is a sundae, then there is no sundae," she sang. Our cups were empty. She licked a bit of chocolate off her fingers.

"Then there is! Come payday. I think we've found a path to enlightenment, Maggie."

"Let's go to your apartment and meditate on it." She looked me steadily in the eyes.

"But I came to your apartment to get away from my apartment. Cliff and Marla are there, and I don't know who all else. Let's go back to your place."

"But I thought you came to rescue me from my place. Those are Josie's friends, and they won't leave. They never leave. I love 'em, and all, but I'm fed up with their company. Nothing against Josie, you understand. She's like a sister."

By then, we'd stepped outside and were standing under a fizzing fluorescent light. Someone inside began turning off the interior lights. Then, the big ice cream cone sign went dark. The gusting wind had grown cold-edged. It nipped at our ears, but we were young, and didn't mind the chill.

"Where, oh, where shall we go?" I asked.

"We could try Christine's. She's been purifying, so nobody's been going around her. Not that she has much company in the first place, since she got dumped. She might like some company. With her, we could have an interesting conversation about something. You'd really like talking to her, Rich. She's been to Mexico, and Peru, and I don't know where all. She knows about things."

"Purifying?"

"Yes. Cool, huh?"

"I guess so. What is it?"

"Flushing out the toxins through strict diet, and meditation. She's preparing for a life-direction change. She'll tell you about it."

"Sounds cool. Lead the way, Maggie."

Maggie took evening classes at the Community College, and had taken an Introductory Anthropology course from Christine. They'd become friends. Christine was five or six years older than us, in her mid-to-late twenties. I'd seen her once or twice at Maggie's apartment. She had an east coast accent, I'd noticed. Maggie clearly admired her, and referred to her often in conversation.

As Maggie told it, when she'd met her, Christine had recently broken up with the man she'd come to Richmond with, and needed a friend. The man (whose name I never learned) had taken a position as an assistant professor in the English department at Richmond's Earlham College. Her anthropological interests had taken her to far-flung quarters of the world. She'd met him in Mexico, and he'd gone along with her to Greece, then Kenya, and then she'd gone with him to Boston, where he'd put the finishing touches on his Masters Degree. When he'd accepted the position at Earlham, she'd welcomed the chance to be still for a while in a quiet Midwestern town in the U.S. "And then he dumped her," Maggie had told me, but when she told the whole story, or as much as she knew, it hadn't been quite that simple.

Then There Is No Mountain

After only six months at Earlham, an offer he had been negotiating, off and on for two years, with a university in Japan, was, finally, formally presented to him. He was thrilled, and wanted to accept it, but Christine refused to go to Japan. He refused to turn it down. They quarreled, bitterly and sadly, for a month, until he'd had to make a decision. He opted to go, and Christine opted to stay. Although they'd made the usual promises to keep in touch, and work things out, somehow, they both knew their relationship wouldn't survive.

"So, how's your mom?" Maggie asked, as we walked. Maggie and I had known each others' families since we were each eight years old. We'd gone to the same Baptist church together, in the small town of Fountain City, ten miles north of Richmond. My mother had been her Sunday School teacher, and her mother had been mine. Her father was a farmer. He and my father had fished together (sometimes on Sunday mornings).

The first time our mothers had caught us kissing out behind the church, they gave us Hell, but we didn't care. The second time they caught us, our mothers began to assume that we'd marry one day. That scared the bejesus out of us both. We never let them catch us again.

We'd each moved from the country to the city, the same summer after high school. She'd gotten a job at the Readmore Bookstore, on Main Street, in Richmond. I walked in one Saturday, looking for "The Travels of Marco Polo," and there she was. We became each other's familiar face (and, from time to time, familiar fingers) in the city.

"Mom's good, I guess," I replied. "I haven't seen her in a couple of weeks. No news is good news. Yours?"

"Mom and Daddy bought forty acres up by Whitewater. They're getting ready to move."

"That's good land up there, I hear."

"Yeah, Daddy says it was at a good price. It's got a creek, and a woods, and it came with a nice, big, old two-story house, too."

We walked for twenty blocks. By the time we got there, we were a little out of breath, and warm, despite the wind.

"I don't see her car," Maggie said. Christine had a ground-floor apartment in a big, converted Victorian house. Several knocks went unanswered. "Follow me." Maggie led me around to the side of the house. We stopped outside a window, the bottom sill of which was about level with our chins.

"Maggie!" I cried, as I understood what she had in mind.

"It's okay! She told me she leaves this window unlocked in case she ever locks herself out. Lift me onto your shoulders."

"Maggie, no. This is breaking and entering."

"No, it isn't. Christine and I are close friends. I have permission."

"You have permission to crawl in her window?" I looked around to see if we were being watched.

"We have an unspoken understanding, okay? That's how close we are."

I just looked at her.

"It's getting cold," she pointed out. She was shivering a little. "Do you really want to walk all the way back to your place?"

I sighed, bent down, and lifted her up onto my shoulders. Her blue-jeaned thighs clutched at my ears as she leaned forward and raised the window. She crawled through it, and closed it behind her. I walked around to the front door. Once she'd let me in, I locked the door behind us.

"I bet she'll be home soon," Maggie guessed, "since she's purifying. It's getting kinda late, so, yeah." She went into the kitchen. I heard glasses clinking and the tap come on.

The room was lit by a lamp at one end of a big, red sofa. A poster of a photo of Jack Kerouac having a smoke on a balcony in New York City was pinned to the wall above a book case stuffed haphazardly with books. Two small African-looking sculptures sat at opposite ends of the book case's top shelf. A framed black and white photo of Christine and a tall bearded man, posing on a mountaintop, stood on one of the end tables. On the wall opposite the Kerouac poster was a poster of a Picasso print–two hands holding a bouquet. Across the room, another case held a stereo system, a small collection of albums, and a collection of clay bowls of different sizes, painted with strange designs. Above that case was a poster of the Mayan calendar.

The book case held books by authors whose names I recognized, but most of whose works I hadn't yet read. Ginsburg, Kerouac, Burroughs, Whitman, Kesey, Heller, Bowles, Didion, Woolf, Roth, Kafka, and others. There were also names I didn't recognize, like Camus, Hesse, Greene, Mead, Leakey, Campbell and Gaddis.

I hungrily scanned the shelves. Titles mixed together like alphabet soup: For Whom The Bell Tolls, The Kama Sutra, Atlas Shrugged, The Kinsey Report. There was a book about mountain climbing, a book about sailing, a book about the joy of sex, and a book of Chinese woodblock prints, which I riffled through, looking for English words, and finding none. The bottom shelf had been reserved for much-used-looking textbooks about anthropology.

The absent Christine, as the owner of all these books, was like a messenger, it seemed to me, from the larger world. I wanted to read every page of every book. I wanted to get the message. A paperback book of poems by someone named Gary Snyder lay on her big, round coffee table.

Maggie had come back from the kitchen with a glass of water for me. She handed it to me, slipped off her shoes, and settled onto on the sofa. I sat down beside her. I drank my water down in one long drink. "Hey, Maggie," I said quietly, after I'd set the glass on the table.

"What?"

"Let's purify." I looked at her sideways.

She smiled. "That's the best offer I've had in a while."

"What do we have to do?"

"I'll ask Christine when she gets here."

"Okay." We sat side-by-side, gazing at the Mayan calendar on the wall opposite.

"Hey, Maggie."

"What?"

"Remember when we used to play hide-and-seek in the cornfields?"

"Yeah."

"A kid can really hide out in an eighty-acre cornfield."

"Yeah. Remember the time we got lost in Daddy's big field?"

"You were so scared."

"So were you."

I picked up the book of poems, and thumbed randomly to a poem which, twisting around to the lamp light, I read to Maggie:

Clambering up the Cold Mountain Path,
The Cold Mountain trail goes on and on:
The long gorge choked with scree and boulders,

Then There Is No Mountain

The wide creek, the mist-blurred grass.
The moss is slippery, though there's been no rain
The pine sings, but there's no wind.
Who can leap the world's ties
And sit with me among the white clouds?

I set the book back on the table, handling it carefully, as if it were breakable, and placed it as precisely as I could onto the spot where I'd picked it up from.

"Huh," I said.

"Huh," Maggie agreed. Neither of us could think of anything else to say.

"It seems late. I'm getting sleepy."

Me, too."

Christine

When I woke up, in Christine's bed, with Maggie sleeping on my shoulder, a whisper of gray light framed the bedroom window shade. It took me a minute to recall Maggie and me waking up in a tangle on the sofa during the night. She'd led me by the hand into the pitch black bedroom. We'd taken off all our clothes, wrapped our limbs around each other under the covers, and made sleepy love before falling back asleep.

I wriggled out of bed, taking pains to not wake Maggie, pulled on my jeans, and, gripping my shirt in my hand, slipped out of the bedroom. Maggie never stirred. As I turned from the bedroom door after carefully pulling it closed, I was jolted by the sight of Christine, simultaneously turning from her front door, her keys in hand, and her eyes widening with surprise when she saw me.

"You're here!" we exclaimed in unison.

"What are you doing here?" she demanded.

"I came with Maggie," I stammered. "We came to see you. She said it would be okay."

"Where is she?"

I jerked my head toward the bedroom door. "Sleeping," I whispered.

She looked at the bedroom door, then back at me, then turned and hung her keys on a hook by the door. It took her a couple of tries to slip the key ring over the hook. Turning back to face me, she put her hands on her hips and looked me up and down. "You sure Maggie's in there?"

I nodded enthusiastically, stepping away from the bedroom door, so she could open it and look in, if she wished.

"How'd you get in?"

"Through the window. Maggie said you'd understand."

"I'm thinking about screaming. Just so you know."

"You'll wake Maggie."

She stifled a smile. "Well, you look pretty harmless. Everyone was wondering where you were," she added, without explanation, as she crossed the room toward her sofa.

"Huh?"

She stopped and turned in front of me, losing her balance slightly as she turned. "I've been at your place all night."

"You've been at my place?"

"I'd heard there was a party there. I was bored out of my mind, so I went." She shrugged, swayed a little, and blinked slowly. "I certainly didn't expect to find you here, in my living room. Shirtless. With your jeans unbuttoned. Not that I was looking for you."

I could feel my face reddening. I changed the subject. "I thought you were purifying."

She smiled at my befuddlement, and then her smile faded. "That ended at midnight. Purification is a lonely business." She glanced darkly at the photo of her and the bearded man on the mountaintop.

I shook my head in disbelief. "We each spent the night at the other's house. And we don't even really know each other. Crazy. So, how was my party?"

She shrugged again. "Loud and long. Lots of boring, intoxicated people. I include myself in that estimation. That Cliff fellow is a train-wreck. Not a happy person, I think. I'd hoped Jacques might be there, stroking his guitar affectionately."

"Jacques was at Maggie's."

She cackled. "That is too much!" She covered her mouth, remembering that Maggie was asleep.

"Well, I was on my way out," I said, after an awkward pause.

"Uh, huh. I need to sit." She lowered herself onto the sofa, and let out a long sigh, followed by a yawn. She closed her eyes.

"I'm just going to get my boots, okay?" They were in front of the sofa, right next to her feet.

"Don't worry. I won't bite." She opened her eyes and regarded me with an amused smirk.

"No, I know, I just—" I knelt, grabbed my boots, and sprang back up to my feet. I was standing close in front of her. "Hey, would you do me a favor?" I blurted, surprising myself.

"What do you have in mind?" Her dark eyes were puffy, and she didn't blink as she stared up at me, waiting. I smelled alcohol wafting up on her breath. She was not the Christine I'd expected to meet. I stepped back.

"Will you be my mom?" I stammered uneasily. My face reddened further. That hadn't come out the way I'd meant it to.

She laughed. "You're a sick puppy. Cute, but sick."

"I'm not really sick," I quickly explained. "I just need to call *in* sick. I really can't work today. I just can't. Would you talk to my boss for me? Tell him you're my mom?"

"Are you joking?" She rolled her eyes.

"Never mind. You don't have to. Dumb idea. I don't know what I was thinking." I shrugged helplessly.

She took a breath, and her smile returned. "Dial it."

"Really?"

"Dial it, before I sober up."

"Ask for Doug," I whispered, once I'd dialed my work number and handed her the phone. "And tell them I have laryngitis." I put on my shirt and boots, and listened as she talked to my employer.

"Hello? May I speak with Doug, please? Yes, this is Mrs. Higgs. Richard's mother. No, yes, no, he's fine. He'll be fine, I mean, once his fever breaks. Well, thank you, dear. We're very proud of him. May I speak with Doug now, please?" Then, after a pause: "Hello? Is this Doug? Good morning, Doug. Mrs. Higgs. I'm afraid Richard is sick today, and I can't allow him to go to work. He has a fever–and laryngitis.

"I see. I'm so sorry. That is unfortunate, sir. I'm so sorry for the late notice. We'd hoped he'd be recovered by this morning. He actually wanted to go, but I'm afraid I had to put my foot down. It could be contagious.

"What? I'm afraid that's not possible, Doug." She held the phone away from her ear for a moment, and I heard Doug's familiar squeaky rant.

"Well, it won't do any good for him to come to the phone," she interrupted his rant. "The boy has laryngitis. I believe I told you that, Doug. I'd have to get him out of bed. Well, since you insist."

She laid the phone on the table. I reached for it, but she waved me away, and placed a finger to her lips for silence. "Richard! Son!" she called out. "Your boss wants to speak with you!" After several seconds, she picked up the receiver. "Here he is, Doug." She set it down again. We heard Doug's excited squawk. After a minute or so, it stopped, and then, after a few more seconds, she picked it up and spoke.

"Hello? Doug? Are you satisfied now? Yes, of course he was there. No, I have no idea what he was saying. I couldn't hear him either. The boy has laryngitis. Do you not know what that means? You do? Then you understand. All right, then. I imagine he'll be fine by tomorrow. Thank you. Thank you. I accept your apology. No, I understand. Yes, I'll tell him once he wakes up again. Have a good day, sir."

"Wow!" I exclaimed, once she'd hung up. "You're amazing."

"Your boss is sorry you're sick, and he wishes you a speedy recovery, because if you don't show up on time tomorrow, you're fired. He asked me to convey that message."

I snorted, dismissing the threat. Doug had threatened to fire me a dozen times in the year that I'd worked for him as a delivery driver. He and his family ran a tobacco, candy, and restaurant supply wholesale business. I delivered to their customers—restaurants and retail stores—in all the surrounding towns, and their customers liked me. I worked for minimum wage, plus all the candy I could pilfer. If he ever did fire me, I wouldn't be losing much, since I was always broke long before payday. Minimum wage jobs were easy to find. Knowing that I could replace them easier than they could replace me enabled me to negotiate our employer-employee relationship from a position of strength. That kind of power had a price, though. The price was poverty. Poverty was my most marketable skill at the time.

"Now, leave, please," Christine ordered. "I can't stay up a minute longer. Out! I have to get myself into bed, now." She rose laboriously to her feet.

"Maggie's in for a surprise when she wakes up." I snickered on my way to the door.

Christine laughed, too, quickly and quietly, as she pushed the door shut behind me. I heard it lock with an emphatic double-click.

Cliff

The sky was still turning blue as I walked away from Christine's door. The air was crisp. I walked briskly, passing by the monolithic County Courthouse, and the old brick Public Library, back to my neighborhood, and, with slowing steps, back to my apartment. I dreaded walking into my living room. I had, for some time, been feeling disassociated from my apartment, and all its clutter, as if it were someone else's place, someone else's clutter. And that someone else had been waiting, with growing impatience, for me to vacate.

To counter the dread on my walk from Christine's, I conjured up my imaginary white room with the white-sheeted sleeping pad against a wall, but the more fully I imagined it, the more cluttered it also became. What about my books? I asked myself. A few of my books might be nice, I conceded. I pictured a row of my favorite paperbacks lined along the base of the wall, with a brick at each end. What about a cross above the bed? I pictured a small, Mexican-style cross of black-painted wood, embellished with silver and little shards of mirror—just that one small, ornate thing against all that white. That would look very cool. But wouldn't it be wrong, to hang a meaningful religious symbol over my bed, just for decoration? It would be disrespectful, at the very least, I decided. No cross, then. But what about my candle in its Chianti bottle holder, for whenever I had a girl over? And what about my records? And something to play them on? I loved my records, so I struggled to accommodate them, a stereo system, and the candle, into my vision, without creating clutter. The fantasy became too complicated. Before I'd arrived at my real apartment, I'd slammed the door on my imaginary one, and returned to the streets where I walked, denied a haven, even in my imagination.

Cliff was sitting on my sofa, where I'd last seen him. He didn't acknowledge me when I walked in. Marla was asleep in a fetal curl beside him. Her face was streaked with black mascara. My apartment was a predictable wasteland of bottles and sacks, cigarette ashes, pizza crusts, smashed potato chips, and smears of unidentifiable matter. The air was heavy with the smell of stale smoke. I sat down in my wingback chair. Cliff had been staring blankly at the chair, and then he stared at me with the same disinterested look.

"You two have to leave," I told him. Somehow, without moving a muscle, without looking away or blinking, he changed his expression from indifference to disdain.

Marla woke up at the sound of my voice. Rising, she asked, "Did somebody make coffee?"

"No! No coffee," I answered, a bit loudly. "I have to get ready for work, and I'm running late. Come on, guys. Out. I don't have much time."

"We got no place to be," Marla replied, stretching suggestively. "After coffee, we'll just stay here and clean up this mess for you, and then go. Okay?"

"We'll lock up for you when we leave," Cliff intoned. "Go ahead, kid. Get ready, and go to work. We'll be fine."

"Get out! This is my house! Seriously. I need some damn privacy. And, what happened to that jailbait you had with you last night?"

"Janis? Oh, she left a long time ago. Looked around, she was gone." Cliff shrugged, mostly with his eyebrows. Neither of them made any attempt to rise from the sofa.

"I thought you were watching out for her," I said to Marla. "You better go find her." Marla looked down at her hands, and said nothing.

"We're more concerned about you, Rich," Cliff said. "You seem depressed, lately. You've been spending a lot of time alone." His cold gaze held me captive. I *had* been spending a lot of time alone. And refusing to answer the door, as often as not.

"I have to have some time to think now and then. What's so bad about that? I've been reading."

"Castaneda?"

"Among others."

"He's a fraud."

"You need friends," Marla said. "We're your friends." She attempted a friendly smile, unaware of the mascara streaking down her cheeks. I shuddered inside.

I ignored his remark about Castaneda. "I'll tell you something else, Cliff. I'm not the one who's depressed. That's you. I'm just frustrated. I mean, last night. You came in uninvited, and threw a party in my living room. I ended up being the one who left–and I live here! I went to Maggie's, to get away from everybody, but Maggie wanted to get away from everybody *there* by going to Christine's, and Christine wasn't home because she was *here*—because she'd heard I was having a party, and that Jacques might be here, but Jacques was at Maggie's! I'm sick of it. Sick of it all, sick of *us* all. I'm always broke two days before payday. Nobody ever talks about anything but scoring dope and getting laid, and who's OD'd, and whose put out a new album, and what's on TV, and blah, blah, blah. It just doesn't add up to anything. Is this really all that's going to happen to us?"

Cliff snorted. "A fine rant, kid. You should feel better, now."

"Stop calling me kid. And leave."

"But, seriously, Rich, do you really think this is all supposed to 'add up' to something? It won't. It never has, and it never will. Hate to burst your bubble, kid."

Marla glared at Cliff, suddenly angry. "Don't start that depressing shit again, you son of a bitch. Everything isn't meaningless, not to me, anyway, just to you, you prick. Stop talkin' like that." She twisted away from him, and hid her face, when he turned his disinterested gaze on her. He watched, unmoved, as she wiped away an angry tear, further smearing her mascara.

"Get out," I said.

He smiled at me. "I'm trying to save you. You're an idealist. Idealism is dangerous. It leads to cynicism—just as sure as pot leads to heroin. Every cynic started out as an idealist. *Don't let it happen to you.*" He smirked as he imitated an anti-drug public service announcement.

"The only thing pot leads to is tooth decay. Any fool knows that." I ignored his real point, which I didn't understand, or care to explore.

"That's funny. Good one. But are you sure about that? Are you ready to test yourself? Try some heroin with me. It's nirvana, friend, like the best pot imaginable, and then even better. Let's try a little. No charge." His eyes glittered dangerously.

"Come on, Cliff," Marla butted in. "I need a cup of coffee. Let's go find some. Let's get some fresh air." Cliff ignored her.

What was I going to have to do to get them to leave? I had an idea. It had worked before, with others. "Well, I got shit to do," I said.

I stood up, went to the stereo, and rummaged through my albums until I found Hank Williams. With practiced swiftness, before they could see who it was, I put on "Lost Highway" and turned it up loud. Then, acting as if they weren't there, I went around the room, gathered empty bottles, and took them into the kitchen. I ran soap and water into the sink, scraped plates and stacked them. I made a couple more trips into the living room to gather bottles and trash. When Marla asked, "What is this hillbilly shit?" I pretended not to hear her over the music. When Cliff asked, angrily, "You remember how ol' Hank died, you dumb country hick?" I just clamped my mouth shut and returned to the kitchen with a handful of trash, pleased with myself for having gotten under Cliff's skin. "This is the same shit-kicker shit my old man listens to!" he yelled over the music.

Cliff hated his father, and his father hated him. Once, I'd gone with him to his parents' house to get his laundry. Their living room was darkened by heavy drapes, on a sunny morning. His father sat enthroned in his easy chair, in robe and slippers, in a pool of yellow lamplight. He folded a newspaper in his lap, and lowered his reading glasses to his chest, where they hung by a chain. There was a lamp table on each side of the chair. On one table was a full brass ashtray with a lit cigarette, curling smoke, a TV guide, a wad of tissue paper, and an orange peel. On the other was a cup of coffee in a chipped saucer, a sugarbowl, a carton of half-and-half, a pack of cigarettes, and a Zippo lighter.

Cliff and his father glared silently at each other as we waited for Cliff's mom to bring him his laundry. The hostility felt as suffocating, and potentially explosive, as a gasoline mist. When his mom came into the room and handed Cliff a laundry bag full of clean clothes, she didn't look any of us in the eye. Cliff thanked her. She told him that was alright, and called him son when she said it, and then left the room. Cliff and his father locked eyes for a moment, and then we left. On our way back to Cliff's apartment, he called his father all sorts of bad names.

Earlham College Incognito

As I washed my dishes, I heard Marla call out, "We're leaving! Bye!" After a minute I peeked into the living room, and confirmed that they were gone. I turned down the music, but I didn't turn it off. My parents loved Hank Williams, and so did I. I'd been listening to his songs all my life. They were as familiar to me as our clothes on the line. I put water in my coffee pot, and coffee in the percolator basket, and set it on the stove. By the time I'd finished washing dishes, the coffee was ready. I turned the record over, sat down on the sofa with a cup, and sipped it slowly.

Once I'd emptied my cup, and the record had ended, I rose and went to the bedroom to change clothes. Janis popped up from the covers in my bed. She lifted my sheet to cover her teenage breasts.

"Jesus Christ!" I swore. "You scared me half to death! What are you doing here?" I demanded.

"I don't know! Where am I?" Her voice was shrill with fear.

I realized I was silhouetted in the doorway, so I stepped to one side. "It's me, Rich. You're in my apartment. It's time for you to go."

She just looked at me dumbly. From the confused look on her face, I gathered that she was still trying to piece together where she was and how she'd gotten there.

"Up!" I barked. "Up and out!" She flinched and raised the sheet to her chin, covering her narrow shoulders. Then I noticed her clothes in a pile by the side of the bed. I went back to the living room and waited in my chair for her to come out. "Keep walking," I ordered, when she hesitated in the bedroom doorway. Her clothes were wrinkled and badly buttoned. Her hair was a mess.

"Where's Marla?" she asked timidly.

"I have no idea."

She was so unsteady on her feet as she headed for the front door, that I relented, and told her to sit down. She dropped onto the sofa instantly, and sat up straight and prim, waiting for further instructions.

"Wait there," I sighed. I went to the kitchen, poured her a cup of coffee, and brought it to her. "Drink this and go."

She held the cup in both hands, took a sip of the bitter, black medicine, made a face of disgust, took another sip and set the cup carefully on the coffee table. "Did we do anything?" she asked, staring meekly into the cup.

"God, no. Finish your coffee."

She sighed with relief, then forced down another sip. "I'm hungry," she murmured.

I had no intention of feeding her. "No food here."

"I'm really hungry."

"If I feed you, you'll come back."

She promised that she wouldn't, not ever. I scrambled my last four eggs, fried two slices of spam, and made toast by suspending the bread over the burner on a fork. While breakfast cooked, I studied the calendar on my kitchen wall. The calendar had a picture of the Smoky Mountains National Park in autumn. Ribbons of morning mist interleaved between the colorful hills.

"Thank you," she said, with a smile that made her look like a little kid for a moment, as I set her plate down in front of her. The food and coffee seemed to revive her, although neither of us said much as we ate. She swallowed her last bite, washed it down with the last of her coffee, and stood up.

She ran her fingers through her hair in an effort to comb it. "I have to find Marla," she said.

"Listen to me, Janis. If you do find out where Marla went, run in the opposite direction, and don't look back. That's all I got to say."

She didn't answer. She just left. I put the dishes in the sink, washed my face, combed my hair, put on clean clothes, and stepped outside, locking the door behind me, and testing it twice.

I walked downtown, passing the library, the courthouse, and the jail, and took the bridge over the Whitewater River gorge. Halfway across the bridge, I paused, as I usually did, to look down at the busy, flashing river two hundred feet below, and the brick ruins of the old Starr piano factory down along the river bank. Two logos, painted onto the bricks, were both still readable, although badly faded: Starr Pianos, and Gennett Records.

Once I'd crossed the river, I walked on, to the brick-and-ivy campus of Earlham College, a place I loved, and a place I'd been going to hide, more and more frequently, in the last few months.

In 1806, thirteen years before Indiana's statehood, Quakers settled just east of the Greenville Treaty boundary, which had been negotiated with Indians in 1795 by General "Mad Anthony" Wayne. The Quakers picked a site near the east bank of the Whitewater River. Their settlement took root and, in 1818, they incorporated it. They named it Richmond. These Quakers were industrious, their fields were fertile, and their frontier town well-placed. They established trade routes, and Richmond continued to prosper and grow. In 1847, they established Earlham College, west of the river.

When I was growing up in the countryside around Richmond, in the 1960s, Earlham College's picturesque brick and ivy campus represented to me the ideal of a temple of learning. Richmond was by then a small city of about 35,000, and a factory town. My father commuted in from the country every weekday to work in a school bus factory.

Then There Is No Mountain

After I'd graduated high school and moved to Richmond, I sometimes walked over to Earlham's Beech-and-Maple-shaded campus to spend an afternoon. I smiled to myself as I walked among the students there. No one could tell that I wasn't one of them. We were the same age, after all. I didn't even have to try to dress like them. Since I was a genuine young proletarian, it was they who tried to dress like me.

I yearned to be one of them. They were smart, I assumed, and they were learning amazing things, I was sure. I would have betrayed myself as a pretender as soon as I spoke to any of them, so I kept quiet, and kept my smile, and my yearning, to myself. I couldn't sit in classes with them, and I couldn't eat with them in their dining hall, so I sat on benches along the walkways in the commons, reading paperbacks. I visited the campus bookstore, where I caressed the merchandise, and I loitered in the student lounge, where I leafed through strange magazines, and eavesdropped on conversations. What prevented me from enrolling, and becoming one of them? A complicated mix of factors, none of which belie the fact that, in the end, I chose not to.

I'd been a pretty good student at Westmont High School, in the isolated farming town of Hollansburg, Ohio, about 25 miles northeast of Richmond. I could have made straight As (my teachers assured me), but B+ had been my favorite grade, right in my comfort zone: better than most, but not the best. That's what I generally tried for, and usually achieved—only occasionally overreaching into A territory. One thing I'd learned in high school was the word "potential", defined as that thing which I wasn't living up to. Nevertheless, I'd enjoyed learning, hungered for it, even, from those of my teachers who'd enjoyed teaching.

Neither my parents, nor their parents, had even considered going to high school. My older brother had gone to high school, but hadn't graduated. My parents knew of no one up either branch of our family tree who'd ever gone to college. They considered it quite an accomplishment when I graduated from Westmont, with a solid B+ average, along with my 38 classmates.

My going on to college was something they were certainly in favor of, if I could figure out a way, but they were in no position to help me. Not by example, not with advice, and certainly not with money. They also couldn't help me with the bewildering, tedious, and voluminous paperwork necessary to select a school, apply, enroll, and secure grants and loans. The inquiries I made (Ohio State, Indiana University, The University of Hawaii, and Earlham College, among others) resulted in thick packets stuffing our mailbox–packets filled with forms, questionnaires, applications, demands that I account for myself. What were my accomplishments? What were my goals? How much money did we have? What were my test results? My interests? My income? My father's income? Where was the supporting documentation for my claims of poverty, athletic excellence, academic prowess, extra-curricular activities, kindness to children?

When I came to understand that a college education is not an end itself, but a means to an end (that end being a chosen profession), it created paralyzing confusion within me. Going to college just to learn about interesting things wasn't the point. Every adult with whom I'd discussed college had assured me I'd have to *choose something* to study in college so that I could then *do* it afterwards, for the rest of my life. If I was smart, and worked hard at my chosen profession, I would probably get rich, they assured me, once I'd paid back all the loans.

But what if, I asked myself, I get a degree, enter my chosen profession, and find out that I don't like it? That I'd made the wrong choice? After all the time, effort, and money invested, I'd be stuck, wouldn't I? To get out, I'd have to choose again, and start over, beginning with the paperwork. And, I'd still have to pay off all the loans.

Had I been sufficiently decisive and motivated, I'd have risen to it. Countless others had done so. However, pulling at me from below the surface, pulling me back down, was an unspoken, but deep-seated, self-imposed, class consciousness at work inside me. College was for the children of other families, rich families. The sums involved in securing a college degree were beyond my comprehension, and the reward too far in the future. So, in my secret identity, on stolen afternoons, I surreptitiously breathed the intoxicating air of higher education, but didn't eat its nourishing food. It was pathetic, really.

Then There Is No Mountain

That afternoon, as I sat sunning on a campus bench, I had an epiphany: I needed a vacation! And in the clarity of that moment, I knew just where I wanted to go. My heart raced with anticipation, as I hiked back across the river. The next day was payday, and I planned go straight from work to the Greyhound bus station and buy a ticket.

The Little Pigeon River

On my way home, I stopped at the library, where I perused their collection of old 78 rpm records. They had an extensive collection of old Gennett recordings. The Gennett recording studios and record pressing plant, which had evolved out of the Starr Piano works down in the gorge, had been an important nexus of the recording industry in the 1920s, and '30s. Some of the musicians who came there to record included Charley Patton, Big Bill Broonzy, Coleman Hawkins, Blind Lemon Jefferson, Jellyroll Morton, Louis Armstrong, Hoagy Carmichael, Duke Ellington, Gene Autry, Uncle Dave Macon, and Guy Lombardo. I'd become a regular at the library, working my way through their Gennett collection, listening intently, trying to develop a coherent overview of the various strains of American music as they branched out from the blues. In addition to the Gennett collection, the library also had a good sampling of the Smithsonian and Folkways catalogs. I spent that afternoon listening to Uncle Dave Macon, Blind Lemon Jefferson, and Woody Guthrie. And speculating about Christine, and her world. And what she might look like naked.

I've always been a non-smoker, but, the next day, I bought a pack of cigarettes on the way to work, and smoked two. I forced myself to inhale the smoke, and suffer through the coughing fit that followed. Doug began to scold me when he saw me, but cut it short when he saw my puffy, red eyes and heard my hoarse voice. Little John caught my eye from across the warehouse.

"Great party," he said later, as we were loading my delivery truck. "Where'd you go? Hey, have you heard the new Moody Blues record yet?"

"No. I hate Moody Blues."

"Right. What about the new Zappa?"

"Haven't heard it. How is it?" We continued to talk about the current music scene while we stacked boxes for delivery into the back of the truck.

At the end of the day, I gathered my meager paycheck, went to the bus station and bought a round-trip ticket to Gatlinburg, Tennessee, a place I'd never been. I told no one where I was going. Next morning, I packed a change of clothes into my backpack, walked to the station and got on the bus. I settled into comfortable anonymity among the other passengers, and looked out the window as we rolled south.

The hills of southern Indiana and Ohio are a kind of illusion. A bus trip, for instance, from Richmond to Cincinnati is a trip from flat, open fields into more rugged, wooded hill country. Cincinnati has place names like Mt. Airy, Mt. Echo, Mt. Adams, and Mt. Storm. Your eyes tell you that you're moving up into the hills from the prairies. However, the elevation of Mt. Airy is a little over 800 feet above sea level. The elevation of Richmond is listed as 981 feet. You are actually moving *down* into the hills–down to the Ohio River basin. When the glaciers had pushed south in the last ice age, over what is now central Indiana, Ohio, and Illinois, they'd scraped the landscape flat. As the glaciers had then receded north to their final puddles, now known as The Great Lakes, meltwater drainage patterns had formed along their southern flanks. Those drainages had become rivers, and the rivers had fed into one massive, transverse drainage ditch, which we call the Ohio River. The rivers draining southward into the Ohio had carved hills out of the slope lowering down to the Ohio Valley. After my bus had crossed the river at Cincinnati, the road pulled us steadily higher, hour after hour, into the Appalachian Mountains.

My motel room in Gatlinburg had a tiny deck that cantilevered out over a rushing stream. After tossing my backpack onto the bed I sat out on the deck and listened to the stream's happy song for a few minutes. Later, in bed, I could hear it through my open window.

The next morning I emptied my backpack onto the bed, and, carrying the empty pack, went to the next-door café, where I had eggs over medium, patty sausage, grits (my first taste), a short stack of buttermilk pancakes, and coffee. After breakfast, I stopped at a grocery store, and bought a loaf of bread, a pack of sliced bologna, sliced cheese, a supply of Oreos, a couple of Moon Pies, a couple of 7-Ups, a Snickers bar and a box of Ritz crackers, all of which I stuffed into my pack at the register. Thus provisioned, and without returning to my room, I hiked to up into the Great Smoky Mountains National Park on the road that roughly paralleled the course of the Little Pigeon River upstream. After a couple of miles, I abandoned the road and picked my way beneath the deep, shading canopy, through the laurel understory, the short distance over to the riverbank.

I'd never seen a mountain stream before. The power of all that pure, clean water charging down through rounded boulders, forming deep, clear pools and sparkling falls, thrilled me. It was loud! Loud enough to drown out my thoughts–even my shouts. I set my pack on the bank and climbed around on the boulders for a while, exploring up and downstream. Big and little fish turned in the refracted light down in the deep pools. No one else was around, so I took off all my clothes and jumped into the cold water. I spent the rest of the day boulder hopping, skinnydipping, sunbathing, and snacking. The roar of the river was the only sound.

When the light began to fail, I hiked back down to Gatlinburg. That night I went to a crowded bar, where I sat in the corner and listened to a stringband play old fashioned music. At first, I mistook the music for bluegrass, because of the similar instrumentation, but it wasn't. It was something older than bluegrass, music as old as the hills themselves, it seemed. I'd heard similar music on scratchy old records, but when I heard it live and loud I understood its power and energy for the first time.

Next day, after breakfast, I caught my return bus home. I gazed out the window as my thoughts roamed free.

After my trip, whenever I turned the pages of my calendar, it was like leafing through vacation pictures. I never told anyone about my excursion. I wasn't missed during my short absence. It pulled me out of my doldrums for a while, got me out of my head, and back into the world.

Then There Is No Mountain

But, the old routines returned, and pulled me down again. I began spending more time alone in my apartment, not answering the door, reading, listening to music, smoking pot, lurking around Earlham's campus, missing too much work, and engaging in an unhealthy level of introspection. I became obsessed with the inner workings of my own mind. I looked too deeply within. There were dark branching hallways, with ever smaller locked rooms deep inside, the contents or occupants of which I couldn't make out clearly, as I pressed my inner eye to damp keyholes, but I saw enough to become deeply frightened on a few occasions.

Into the Dark

One evening, during the last page of my calendar, after pacing anxiously back and forth in my apartment for I didn't know how long, I walked, through a black wind blowing white snow, to Maggie's place. The deep cold was like one long, sweet slap in the face. "Thank God you're home," I sighed, when she let me in. I hadn't seen her in a month. We were alone. Once we'd settled onto her sofa, I pulled a joint from my pocket and offered to share, but she declined, telling me she had quit, probably for good. In fact, she continued, she was glad I'd come over, because she'd wanted to tell me that she was moving back home, meaning back with her parents, into their newly purchased farmhouse. She'd had enough of city life. Her plan was to save up money for the next fall, when she would be entering Indiana University in Bloomington, as a full-time student. She'd given notice at her job in Richmond. She knew she could always wait tables at The Fountain Grille in Fountain City, owned by family friends, for a bit of income between then and the fall. Maybe I'd see her sometimes when I made deliveries there on my route.

By the time she'd told me all this, I'd slipped the joint back into my pocket, and sunk deep into her sofa. She asked me to stay and eat. We had Hamburger Helper and chocolate milk. "I wish the Dairy Queen was open," I mumbled as we ate. "Closed for the season, freezin's the reason," Maggie replied, quoting their icicle-y sign. She smiled, hoping to coax a smile out of me, I could tell, and I couldn't help but smile back at her.

She had to get ready for a movie date. I was welcome to stay after she'd left, she told me, but I rose to go. Before I put my coat on, as we stood by her door, she hugged me tight and long. "Please take care of yourself," she said, and looked me steadily in the eyes to let me know she meant it.

I pushed through the bleak night, back to my place, and slammed my door shut behind me. Ah, Maggie. The rest of the evening, I suffered through a meltdown, until, exhausted and dulled, I finally fell asleep.

Then There Is No Mountain

When, a few days later, I showed up uninvited at Christine's door, it was lanky Jacques who answered the doorbell, squinting into the brilliant winter sunlight, which was intensified by fresh, deep snow. He didn't know me, but the temperature outside was only 10 degrees, so, when I asked if Christine was home, he had to decide quickly whether to let me in, or send me away. He ushered me in. The room smelled like chocolate chip cookies. Christine stood in her kitchen doorway, looking at me in surprise.

"Hello, Richard. What brings you here?" she asked. A man with a sandy beard, and a woman wearing a beret, sitting together on the sofa, studied me with interest. Jacques' guitar leaned in a corner. Some cool jazz trumpet played low on the stereo.

I discovered that I was as surprised as her to find myself standing there, dripping a puddle onto her floor. In my over-heated imagination, I must have expected her to be alone. I quickly made up and uttered a lie about wanting to borrow a book.

"Which book?" she wanted to know, reasonably.

"That one with the poems about the cold mountain," I stammered. It was the only one that came to mind, even though I hadn't thought about it again until that moment.

She told me she was happy to lend it to me. She asked me if I wanted to warm up "for a minute" before I left.

"Can't stay," I replied.

As she placed the book into my hand, she briefly covered my cold hand with her warm one. "Keep it," she said. "Wait a minute," she added, as I thanked her and turned to go. She went to the kitchen, and when she came back, she handed me a cookie on a paper napkin. Jacques opened the door for me. "If you see Maggie, have her phone me," she called out, as Jacques was closing the door.

I crunched through the snow to the top of a small rise at the end of her block, slid into my car, set the cookie and book on the seat, wiped my nose on the napkin, turned on the key, took the car out of gear, released the brake, and began to coast down the street toward the bottom of the hill. Once I had sufficient speed, I slipped it into second gear, popped the clutch, and the engine started. My starter hadn't worked for months. Parking on hills, and popping the clutch to start my car, had become second nature.

What had I wanted from Christine? Everything. Salvation. Succor. Suggestions. Sex. All at once. What had she given me? A cookie and a poem. Hard times. I ate the cookie on the way home, although I can't say I enjoyed it. The book of poems went onto my shelf, unopened.

That winter seemed as if it would never end. Gray snow piled up, plowed into furrows along frozen streets, white steam rose from buildings, rusting cars refused to start. I studied the works of Carlos Castaneda, Woody Guthrie (from the library), and Vincent Van Gogh (whose paintings were featured on my new calendar.)

I sometimes went to parties on weekends, in overheated rooms, with coats piled in corners, music blaring, and smoke drifting. I sometimes brought young women home. I remember their sweet, flushed faces, nested in furry collars. Their busy eyes looking around my room as their fingers came out of their mittens, and they opened their coats. My melancholia inevitably drove them away. I could be fun, but not for very long.

Cliff seemed to have moved into other circles. The few times I saw him, Marla wasn't with him. The last time I saw him, he'd lost weight, and teeth, and seemed to vibrate with nervous, violent energy. By Spring, he'd disappeared, along with the snow, and word spread that he was in jail. No one knew the details, but no one was surprised.

On my twentieth birthday, in April, my mom and dad knocked on my door, to my surprise. They declined to come in. Instead, they stayed on the doorstep, and invited me out to their place for birthday cake. "Okay," I replied. "About what time should I come out?"

"You can follow us out there right now, if you want to," Mom said.

"Okay." I got my keys and came outside. I was surprised by how glad I was to see them. I'd been avoiding them for months.

When Dad saw that I was parked a half-block away at the top of a slope, he asked, "You still ain't got that starter fixed yet?"

"Starters cost money, Dad."

He just nodded. As I was following them out of town, he pulled into a parts store. I parked on the highest point in the parking lot, by habit, but I knew I wouldn't have enough slope to restart the car, so I set the brake, left the engine running, and hoped it wouldn't die. Dad had already gone inside when I got to the door. "What are you doing?" I asked him as he strolled up to the waiting clerk at the counter. He just glanced at me without answering. To the clerk, he said, "I need a starter rebuild kit for a '62 Belair."

"V8?"

"Yep. 283."

"Just a minute."

Once he'd paid for the kit, he handed it to me. "Happy birthday, son."

That afternoon, in his driveway, we crawled under my old Chevy together, and unbolted the starter. Then, he sat on a lawn chair on the concrete patio pad by his front door, smoking cigarettes, and talked me through disassembling the starter. I sat cross-legged on the patio, at his feet. Then, he talked me through rebuilding it, using the parts from the kit.

"You got to hold that spring back the whole time," he said. "No. Not like that. Don't be so impatient. You can do it, son. Watch your fingers." His own fingers, pantomiming as he talked, had permanent brown stains from a lifetime of holding cigarettes. "Damn. Well. Try her again. Yep. Yep. That's the way." Whenever I looked up at him, he smiled at me, deepening the lines on his familiar old face. "Now, spin it. Yep. That ought to work." We crawled back under the Chevy and remounted the starter.

Working together was all we needed, to remind ourselves how we felt about each other, so we didn't talk about much, except the task at hand. He was that way with all his sons. We grinned at each other when, later, I turned the ignition, and the engine fired up. "We probably ought to've done the solenoid, too," he said, "but I reckon she's okay for now."

As evening came, my brothers and sister began to arrive. Mom made fried chicken. Then we had cake. They all sang to me, and I blew out the candles. I got a bottle of Brut aftershave lotion from each of my brothers, and another one from Mom and Dad. My sister gave me a gold-plated toothpick in a little case, as a joke. I was twenty years old. Mom gave me a sentimental card. "Now, don't be such a stranger, son," she scolded. "We like to see you now and then."

And then, the best thing happened: it was no longer about me. We all spent the rest of the evening kidding each other, reminding each other of our stories, and advising each other on the ways of the world. When I got back to my apartment in town that evening, with my armload of aftershave lotions, and my toothpick, and my card, and a big piece of leftover cake, I set everything down on my dining room table, and looked around. I went from room to room. Everything was familiar. Nothing seemed like mine. I looked into the bathroom mirror, but quickly looked away, as if a stranger had caught me staring. I sat on the sofa, and said, out loud, "Something has to change. You need to make a plan."

Yes, Rainier!

Many years later, as I sat in the sun recovering from surgery, in my Tulsa backyard, the book of Cold Mountain poems fell from my hands, when I was startled out of my reverie by the clank and squeak of my backyard gate. It was Joe, come to have coffee with me. After he'd filled our cups and settled into a chair, we sat by the pond, talking about this and that, listening to my little waterfall.

During a lull in the conversation, I said, "Rainier."

Joe smiled, suddenly alert. "Rainier?" he asked.

"Yes, Rainier!" I replied. "I've been thinking." By then, we were both grinning. We spent the rest of the morning talking with growing excitement about the climb—when we should go, and how we should train, once I was fully recovered from surgery.

Eight hard-trained months later, at Whittaker Base Camp in Ashford, Washington, we stood with our newly-formed climb team in a semi-circle around our guides. When it was my turn to introduce myself to my new teammates and say why I'd come there, I kept the story short. I just said, "Well, Joe talked me into it. We've climbed a couple of peaks together, and we just want to take it to another level." I think Joe said something similar.

There were eighteen of us in total. After introductions, we were divided into two groups, each assigned to a different set of guides. We went into The Hut and watched a PowerPoint about Rainier Mountaineering Incorporated, Whittaker Base Camp, Mount Rainier, and their common histories. RMI had been guiding climbers up Rainier since the 1960s.

Joe and I stopped by the rental desk, where I rented oversize hardshell hinged plastic boots with liners, crampons, gaiters, a parka, a helmet, and an avalanche transponder. Joe rented the same except for a parka, which he already owned. Walking in those boots takes some getting used to. You must rent them a couple of sizes larger than your normal boots. Their hard, hinged shells don't flex much as you walk, so, on level ground, you clomp around in them like Frankenstein's monster.

I noticed a board showing conditions at the summit. Fifteen degrees, clear, and a twenty-mile-per-hour wind at last report. There was also a notation of their year-to-date success rate for summiting: 75%. We assured each other that we wouldn't be among the 25% who'd failed. After taking care of business, we whiled away the evening. We had burgers and beer at the outdoor *taverna*, and chatted with some of our new teammates, and with other climbers who were there in different stages of their four- or five-day climbs. RMI operates an assembly line, with a constant turnover of climbers during climbing season. Base Camp is always a beehive of climbers checking in, checking out, heading up, returning down, comparing notes, celebrating or comforting one another, and faring each other well after an intense, shared experience. We shopped in the mountaineering store, and then went back to the room where we compulsively disarranged and rearranged our packs. When it grew dim enough outside, around ten o' clock, I lay down and closed my eyes.

Next morning, our teams assembled at some picnic tables, roll was taken, and our lead guides, Jon Shea and Win Whittaker, went over the day's itinerary. We'd be climbing up to about 6,500 feet, just above the Rainier National Park visitor center at a place called Paradise. We'd spend the day on a snowfield learning basic mountaineering skills. They explained in detail what gear, clothing, and supplies we'd each need to have for our ascent. They covered practical issues, like how much food to pack and what kind, and how much water, and how to pace your drinking. And if you have to pee? Simple. Just wait for a break, if you can, and walk off a ways and do it. And if you have to poop, well, that was simple, too, at least in theory. The guides would be carrying "blue bags," and if you felt the need and couldn't wait, you would simply ask a guide for a blue bag, walk off a ways, take care of business, scoop your poop into the bag, pack the bag into your pack, and rejoin the group, who would be waiting around for you to finish up so everyone could get back to climbing the mountain.

A large-framed older man, who looked to be in his mid-sixties, and whose muddy khakis and tee shirt gave the impression he'd been digging in his garden, strode up to the guides with long, easy steps. They immediately deferred to him, and he introduced himself to us. He was Lou Whittaker, the founder of RMI, and, as proprietor of Whittaker Bunkhouse, our host. A murmur of admiration rippled through the group. Lou Whittaker was the first American to summit Everest from the north face. He'd summitted Rainier 250 times and had trained a couple of generations of mountain guides, who'd in turn climbed, and trained others, all over the world. He didn't talk to us about any of that. He talked to us about making deposits into our fitness banks while we were still young, and to him, we were all young, even me. He'd made regular deposits into his fitness bank for most of his adult life, and now, in his "retirement," he was making withdrawals. He was, he said, living off of his fitness investment. He hoped we'd follow his example. He was eighty years old, he said, and we were amazed.

One of our lead guides was his son Win, and the other, Jon Shea, had just returned from a successful Everest summit a few weeks before. We were in good hands. Our entire crew of guides, about a half dozen, was young, male, laid back, and fit. You couldn't have squeezed a pint of body fat out of their collective selves. They tended to be slender and long-limbed, except for Jon, who was more compact and muscular than the others. We had noticed one female guide the evening before, standing with some other guides in a circle, talking guide-talk. She was as unadorned as her male peers. Although she was shorter and weighed maybe 30 pounds less than any of her colleagues, she radiated physical confidence, as they all did. It was difficult to imagine her in powder and paint under any circumstance, but still, her femininity was undiminished. She seemed like a reminder of a more ancient model of the female, one who ran with wolves, perhaps.

A couple of other things we noticed about our guides: In addition to the usual fashion sense of mountaineers, which tends to involve expensive, nicely detailed layers of manmade materials in bright colors or black, our

103

guides seemed to like white-framed sunglasses. Also, they only wore sandals, except when it was necessary to put on their climbing boots. Once they were off the slope, the boots came off first thing, and the sandals went back on. They all paid a lot of attention to their feet.

We boarded the RMI bus, the guides in their sandals, and the rest of us clomping awkwardly in our oversize Frankenstein boots. During the 30-minute ride through rainforest switchbacks to the visitor center at Paradise, the guides flexed their toes, pulled their caps over their eyes, and napped while the rest of us chattered excitedly. It had begun!

At Paradise's parking lot we disembarked and broke up into two teams. Joe and I went with the team assigned to Jon Shea and another guide, Eric. The others went with Win Whittaker. We were at about 5,500 feet, at the base of Muir Snowfield. We put on light packs and helmets, and, gripping our ice axes, climbed single-file about a thousand feet to the top of a steep snow-covered ridge. There we spent the day learning a few basic mountaineering skills, such as how to kick-step your boots into the steps made in the snow by the person before you, and how to rest-step by locking your back leg at the knee while swinging your foreleg up to the next step. We also learned how to compensate for the high-elevation pressure differential between the air in your lungs and the blood in your arteries by pressure breathing—forcing air out of your lungs through partially pursed lips to create enough back pressure to force more precious oxygen through the capillary walls in your lungs. We also learned how to traverse a steep slope while roped together, how to use our ice axes to do a three-point self-arrest if we fell, and how to do a group self-arrest if someone roped to us fell.

By the end of this day of focused play, we'd acclimated somewhat, gained a modest set of skills and confidence, and gotten to know each other better. We met up with the other group in the visitor center parking lot, the guides all changed into their sandals, and we boarded the bus. The guides napped on the way back to Base Camp, as the rest of us chattered happily about the day's play. Back at Base Camp, the guides presided over a short debriefing and a preview of the next day's plan, after which we dispersed. Next day would be the first leg of our summit attempt. Joe and I were both a little nervous. Our eight months of training and preparations were about to be put to the test. No matter how much we'd done, no matter how much more we could have done, there was nothing left to do but prepare ourselves mentally, go over our gear and supplies yet again, and try to get a good night's rest.

I began to stress over the fact that I had been constipated for several days. What if, God forbid, I had to ask for a *blue bag* halfway up the mountain? I could not allow that to happen. I walked down the street to Ashford's only store, an old-time general store, and bought a packet of Ex-lax. I'd never taken Ex-Lax before so I read the directions carefully. There were two small chocolate-looking bars in the packet. Adults were to take "two chocolate pieces." I decided to only eat one of the bars and put the other one away. My anxiety subsided and I piddled around over the evening, going through my gear, reading on the porch, thinking about the climb, and waiting. I didn't realize that I'd misunderstood the directions. When the laxative hit later that night, it hit hard, in several convulsive waves, lasting until morning. At some point during that long night, I realized something wasn't right, so I reviewed the directions. Each of the bars was divided into eight smaller breakaway pieces. Two of those small pieces were the actual recommended dosage. Not two bars. I'd taken eight pieces, four times the recommendation.

By morning, when it was time to get up and get going, my gut was as empty as a tube of toothpaste that's been run over by a truck. Unfortunately, it was still churning to the point that, empty as I was, it was difficult to eat. I forced down part of a breakfast sandwich, and a cup of coffee, which settled my stomach. Then I got focused on getting ready to climb the mountain. For the umpteenth time, Joe and I sorted through our gear. Then we dressed in our high-tech layers, put on our Frankenstein boots, hoisted our packs onto our backs—*they were heavy!*—and clomped over to the gathering place to join our mates.

There was a quiet hum of excitement about us as we gathered for the briefing. We'd start from the parking lot at the Paradise Visitor Center, as yesterday, and we'd climb in two groups of nine climbers each. Each group would be led by a team of three guides. We'd climb up the Muir Snowfield, past where we'd practiced the day before, and continue up along an established route. We'd climb for an hour or so, rest for ten minutes, climb for an hour, rest for ten minutes, until we got to Camp Muir at just above 10,000 feet. It was expected to take about five hours to reach Muir. Our rests would be brief, because we had far to go, and also, they pointed out, because when we were sitting, we were losing the heat we'd built up while climbing. And it was cold up there. At the breaks, we'd need to get our packs off our backs, get off our feet, drink water in measured amounts from our total supply, eat as much food as we could get down, and be ready to resume climbing when our guides stood up.

Once we'd debussed at the Paradise Parking Lot, the guides changed out of their sandals, took roll call, and the team led by Win took off. Our team, led by Jon Shea, waited ten minutes and followed.

We climbed in a close single file, pressure breathing, rest-stepping into the boot prints of the person before us, and steadying ourselves with our climbing poles. I made it fine to the first break, although I was breathing more heavily than I'd expected. The pack was heavy, and the path was unvaryingly steep. We dug out our water bottles and food items, and sat on our packs in a loose circle, eating and drinking with serious intent, and exchanging small talk between bites. Almost immediately, it seemed to me, the guides then stood up and slung their packs on, which was our cue to do the same. We rose, stowed our water bottles and food containers, got our packs and hardhats on and headed out. I was the last one ready, so I fell in at the rear of the line.

We climbed up into a cloud that girdled the mountain. Visibility dropped to a couple of hundred feet, and then less as we climbed into the thick monotonous gauze. Even our brightly colored clothes were muted by the cloud that enveloped us. There was little talk as we focused on technique to coordinate steps, rests, and breaths for maximum efficiency. The guides had arranged themselves at the head and tail, with a rover in between who observed us and offered advice and encouragement.

The grade grew steeper, and my pack grew heavier. The distance between me and the man before me also grew. I concentrated on technique, efficiency. By the time the next rest was called an hour later, I'd had to stop and breathe a few times for a few seconds, to push oxygen into my lungs, into my blood, out to my muscles, and to let my racing heart slow. At the break, the earliest ones were already sitting on their packs, eating and drinking, when the last of us arrived. I got my pack off, dug out my water and food, and gorged. I spoke little. Breathing was the only thing that mattered between bites and gulps. I had just gotten settled onto my pack, it seemed, when the guides rose to their feet, signaling that the break was over. I was still eating as I rushed to stow my food and water. I stood up, slung my pack on, steadied myself on the poles and turned to get in line. The line had already formed and was already moving. How had this happened so fast? I stepped quickly into the path and caught up, attended by Eric, the rear guide. Soon, I began to fall behind, step by step, as we climbed further into the cloud, which became thicker still. The next rest, an hour later, ended with my teammates suddenly standing ready to go just as I had begun to catch my breath, just as I had begun to replace the fuel and water I'd expended. Joe fell in somewhere in their middle. He was having no trouble keeping pace.

I fell further and further behind the group. Eric became my personal guide, a long-limbed shepherd with one stray, struggling sheep. I focused intensely on technique: swing a foot up and kick it into the snowstep left by the climber before me, lock the back knee to put my weight onto my bones and off my muscles, swing my arms and poles, pressure breathe in synchronized rhythm with my steps, and pull myself up the mountain one step after another. Eric allowed me to set the pace while at the same time urging me upwards with words of encouragement, and reminders of the importance of reaching Camp Muir in time to rest for the final push to the summit. He reminded me to breathe right when I'd forget, and urged me *not to rush* myself but to set and keep a steady pace.

My heart seemed to be frantically trying to find a way out of my rib cage. I couldn't seem to deliver enough power to my legs. I had to stop at regular intervals, rest on my locked back leg and take five or six deep pressure breaths before I could move on. When we finally stopped for a break, still deep in the cloud, it was hard to eat and drink but I choked down what I could, and then sat on my pack, stupefied, motionless, staring into the gauze, breathing with intent.

Eric sat beside me to patiently wait until I could go on. "So, what kind of training did you do to prepare for this?" Eric gently inquired.

I told him that I'd been training steadily for eight months. I'd started out in a gym with a routine of core conditioning exercises, Stairmaster, walking lunges, and yoga classes twice a week. I'd augmented this with outdoor exercise, including trail running and light jogging. About four months before the climb, I'd quit the gym and replaced the Stairmaster work by finding a steep 250 foot hill and climbing it under a weighted pack every Saturday. I started out with 25 pounds in the pack and did three laps. Once I reached 5 laps, I increased the weight to 35 pounds and dropped back to 3 laps. Once I'd reached 5 laps again I increased the weight again. Before long I was climbing six laps packing 47 pounds once or twice every week. About two months prior to the Rainier climb I added jogging twice a week, steadily increasing the distance.

"Well, that sounds good then." His tone implied that my explanation of my training only deepened the mystery of why I was struggling so much. I hadn't mentioned the halt to my aerobic training three weeks before the climb, which was brought on by the mysterious sharp pain in my stomach that lasted several days. I *certainly* didn't tell him that I'd begun that morning stupidly dehydrated and drained of all fuel. I did tell him that I was grateful for him hanging back with me, and for his patience and encouragement.

"Hey, you're doing fine," he replied. "You're hanging tough. We're gonna make it."

"Yes. No question."

"Let's go before we lose any more heat." He sprang to his feet. I struggled to mine.

On our next break, we didn't speak. As I sat there, a bird materialized out of the cloud, landed on my ski pole, looked me over, and flicked away. I became fixated on a spider creeping over the snow. Every breath was an event in itself.

When we climbed up out of the cloud we were in brilliant sunshine. We were above the treeline so the mountain loomed above us composed solely of snow, basalt, and patches of tundra where the snow had been blown clear.

"Can we see the camp from here?" I asked Eric between breaths. I was breathing harder and climbing slower than ever.

He pointed it out, the dark dash of a basalt ridge far above us. Reading my thoughts, he gave me some advice. "It's further than it looks, Richard. We've got a ways to go, so don't fixate on it or you might get discouraged."

Well, we wouldn't want that, would we? I thought. Following his advice, I kept my eyes on the prize, which was nothing but the next step, and the next, and always just one step ahead.

My pace slowed with every step toward camp, ever closer yet ever slower, as if I were acting out one of Xeno's paradoxes. Once, when I had stopped to breathe, Eric said to me, reluctantly, and a bit formally: "At this point, Richard, we have to wonder if you'll be able to continue beyond Camp Muir."

He seemed relieved when I told him I had already decided that Camp Muir was as far as I intended to climb.

It was about 5 p.m. when we joined the rest of the team at Camp Muir. Everyone, Joe especially, was glad to see me. They all patted my back, shook my hand, high-fived me, and told me they were proud of me for not turning back, as had been rumored.

Camp Muir

Camp Muir is cemented and bolted onto a thin basalt ridge that juts up out of the snow, separating the vast Muir Snowfield below from the upper reaches of Cowlitz Glacier. If you have any breath left when you get there, the view will take it away. Its elevation is somewhere between 10,050 and 10,188 feet, depending on which map you consult. Or where you're standing, for that matter. The camp has several buildings, including a crude tarpaper and plywood hut. The hut is about the shape of a boxcar, but smaller. It is walled off into two sections, one for RMI climbers and the other for climbers using another guide service. There's also a stone WPA-style hut provided by the National Park Service for independent climbers. Sitting on a slightly higher section of the ridge is the park rangers' stone hut, outside of which rangers can be seen sitting aloof in the sun reading Edward Abbey while the steady ebb and flow of climbers mills around below their feet. There is also a weather station and several outhouses. Far below us the top of the cloud we'd climbed through still skirted the mountain, although it was beginning to break apart. In the distance we could see Mt. Adams and Mt. St. Helens, and, beyond them, magnificent Mt. Hood. Above us towered the remaining 4,400 feet of Rainier, the summit tucked out of view behind jagged foreground peaks. Above Rainier was the immaculate cold sky, a thin, blue membrane darkened by a deeper darkness beyond.

We were to relax and eat and then get into our sleeping bags by 6:30 and try to sleep. The guides would wake us sometime between midnight and 1:30 a.m. to gear up quickly and head out for the summit attempt. Most of the climb would be in the dark and cold of night. The team would be roped together, and they would light their way by their headlamps. It's necessary to begin at such an ungodly hour so that the summit can be reached by mid-morning at the latest. This allows a team to finish a descent from the summit to the visitor's center by mid-afternoon. We were told that we needed to be off of Rainier before the daily afternoon summer storms visited the upper reaches of the mountain. It wasn't mentioned that we also needed to be out of the hut by mid-afternoon to make room for the next wave of RMI climbers.

By around 5:30 the guides had boiled a five-gallon jug of water. We used the water to pour over our dehydrated meals, and make tea or hot chocolate. We all gathered together in the hut and ate ravenously, cheerfully stuffing our bellies with warmth. After we ate, Joe and I stepped outside. We each looked out toward Mt. Adams to the south.

"What are you gonna do?" he asked, knowing it wasn't necessary to explain what he meant.

"This is as far as I'm going, Joe."

He nodded. "Me, too, bro."

I looked at him in surprise. "Joe. Listen to me. If you're staying back because of me, don't."

"I'm not."

"Because, and I mean this, I won't appreciate it. It will be a wasted gesture."

"I know that."

"Go to the top if you can, Joe. Please. Represent us."

He looked at me finally. "I don't trust myself to go any further."

"Are you sure?"

He nodded.

"I'm sorry, Joe."

"Don't be. Look at this view, bro!" The cloud below us had dissipated. We could see the visitor's center parking lot far below us, and the endless green rainforests spreading out below that over the rugged lowlands, all side-lit by the late afternoon sun. We stood far above it all, in a world of white snow, black basalt, and blue sky. Camp Muir was a fine place to be. We told Jon Shea that we'd be staying in camp. Out of our group of eighteen, we were the only two who had decided to stop there.

The main room inside the hut is composed of two sleeping platforms, one above the other. The platforms are each just an expanse of plywood decking arranged in an L around two walls. The climbers are expected to arrange their sleeping bags side-by-side, and there is just enough room for eighteen climbers. When I went to pick out my spot, I found that every berth had apparently been taken. After surveying the situation for a few minutes I concluded that if I moved two sleeping bags apart at the very end, I could make just enough room for mine between them. After arranging my bed, I went outside until it was time to bed down.

When the time came, I was, as usual, the last person to act. I climbed up to my berth and found a young married couple there, the woman lying where I'd made my bed. "We moved your bag to the end," she explained. "Unless you'd *rather* sleep between us?" she teased.

"Oh, no, no," I mumbled, embarrassed. "Sorry, I didn't know..." The two of them just giggled and returned their attentions to each other. I settled in beside her, but demurely placed my head near her feet and my feet near her head. Then the lights went out.

When the lights came back on, sometime after midnight, I woke and sat up in place to watch all my teammates struggle quietly in the confined floor space, getting around each other and into their cold-weather clothes, and then making their ways out into the black night to continue gearing up. Once the traffic had cleared inside the hut I also got up, dressed, and joined them all outside. Joe, in his berth on the opposite side of the room from me, hadn't stirred. Outside, there wasn't much joking around, as everyone helped each other check and re-check their equipment, supplies, and clothing. The guides moved among them, tightening straps, checking laces, testing head-lamps and avalanche transponders, making sure everyone's carabiners were in order, and all the other necessary things, all the while reminding every-one that there was no time to waste. I stood inconspicuously among them, preparing along with them in my mind, feeling their strange brew of grim excitement. Before long, the guides had arranged them into their two groups.

Win's team left the camp first, roped together for the rising traverse up across steep, bowl-shaped Cowlitz Glacier to Cathedral Gap. Jon's team waited a few minutes. RMI keeps their parties broken up into smaller teams to minimize risk, and also out of consideration to other climbing parties they encounter on the climb. There's also an aesthetic consideration. Smaller par-ties have a smaller visual impact on the mountainside. Jon's team was lined up at the camp's edge, roped together and waiting for the command, like a team of horses.

I was sitting against a rock in my parka looking up at the sky. One of the guides, unaware, or forgetting, that Joe and I were staying behind, padlocked the door to the hut to secure the climbers' bedding and other left-behind items. I was stargazing, so I wasn't aware of what he was doing, but Joe, who'd been awake in his bunk, heard the sound of the door closing, and the latch clapping shut, and understood immediately that he was being locked in. He yelled out, jumped from bed, rushed to the door, and started banging and yelling out to the surprised guide, who immediately unlocked it. If Joe hadn't been awake and alert, he would have spent the night locked in and I would have spent the night locked out. I would have had a long, potentially dangerous night.

As the last team headed out, I watched the silent glowworm line of their headlamps grow smaller, dimmer, and higher in the night. The climb from Camp Muir to the summit is steeper, colder, windier and more treacher-ous than the climb from Paradise to Muir. Every foot you gain delivers less oxygen to your lungs, your blood, your muscles. Making that climb roped together in the deep dark of a moonless night intensifies the danger and dif-ficulty. The real test had begun for them.

I lingered outside the hut once the camp had emptied, and returned my attention to the sky. I'd been looking forward to viewing the night sky from up there for months. Since it was the summer solstice and we were at a fairly high latitude, the evening light didn't drain from the sky until well after 10 p.m. and first light would be around 4 a.m. Darkness would be relatively short-lived. But what a darkness! It also happened to be a new moon, so the mountain was lit only by stars, and at that altitude the stars were sharper and brighter than I'd ever seen them, crowding out the sky. The Milky Way splashed from horizon to horizon. My mind emptied out to the stars, and I contented myself with just looking. I didn't look for anything up there. I just looked. When the time felt right, I went into the hut, burrowed into my sleeping bag, and slept deeply.

At about 4 a.m., I was awakened by the sound of the hut door sliding across the floor as it was being opened, then the sounds of boots and heavy breathing. I sat up. "Who are you?" I demanded. Joe had awakened, too, in his corner, and said, "Hello?" They were three of our teammates from Win's group, who had reached their limit up there and had to turn back. They sat heavily on the edge of the lower platform and undressed by the darting lights of their headlamps. They were in no condition for conversation, but I gleaned from their mutterings that they couldn't keep up the pace required by the guides. Their legs had become unsteady. They'd been exposed to winds of 30 to 40 miles per hour, and the temperature had dropped to 15 degrees. Even in their parkas, if they weren't working, they were freezing, and they could work no more. They hadn't made it to the high break, where the slope relents somewhat for the final push to the rim and summit. One by one their headlamps went out as they crawled, defeated, into their sleeping bags and became silent. I fell back to sleep. Another small group returned a couple of hours later, and then, at about 8 a.m., another. Although each group had made it further than the previous group, they were all in the same state of exhaustion and deep disappointment. In total there were 10 of us who didn't make the summit, out of the 18 who'd signed up. Those who had made it would have been reaching the summit at about the same time the last group to turn back made it back down to Camp Muir.

I got up, dressed, and went outside. Joe came out soon after. We'd been the only ones who'd gotten a good night's sleep, and we were feeling great. It was a beautiful morning with the world at our feet. The thin mountain air was exhilarating. We leaned against the hut facing the sun and had our morning coffee, from a bag I'd filled with whole roasted coffee beans and Hershey's chocolate chips in a fifty-fifty ratio. We each chewed up a tasty mouthful and washed it down with cold water. Two or three mouthfuls were all it took to add a nice caffeine buzz to our mountain-morning high.

We spent the morning idling around camp, taking pictures, chatting with climbers from our group and others. Naturally, we were all disappointed, but for the most part, we'd become philosophical, or at least stoical, about not reaching the summit. However, one of those who had come back during the night, Eileen, a very fit middle-aged pediatrician and university professor from New Hampshire, had invested a lot of her self-esteem into reaching the summit, and couldn't yet suppress her disappointment, her humiliation. She needed to talk about it. It was she who had talked her party into climbing Mount Rainier, she who had led them there, and she the only one among them who'd failed. She'd always been a high acheiver, and in a life full of successes, failure was not a familiar experience.

It seemed to me that climbing Mount Rainier was, for her, not just a measure of her fitness, but also a measure of where she stood in the crowd. We consoled her as best we could. We offered her alternate ways to think about it, as opposed to success/failure, as opposed to summit/failure, and so on. She expressed our own disappointments for us, more or less. We consoled ourselves when we consoled her. Each of us was going to have to accept, and maybe even embrace, our experience on the mountain, regardless of the elevation at which we'd had to turn around. As for me, I'd gone there to find my limit, wherever that was, and I'd found it. I knew I'd gone as far as I could in the time allotted, and I was satisfied with that. More than satisfied, I was grateful. Grateful to Louise for her months of patient support as I'd prepared for the climb, to Joe for not only making it possible, but *insisting* on it, and to Eric, who'd so patiently guided me to my limit.

About mid-morning one of the guides who'd returned invited any of us who cared to go on a short hike to the top of Muir Peak, a smallish spire at the east end of the camp. It was something to do. Four of us joined him. Joe declined. From the top, we were about 150 feet above the camp. We savored the view for a few minutes. I also savored the fact that I had now climbed higher than Joe, something I intended to never let him forget.

Around noon, the first group of our summiteers returned. We gave them a hero's welcome. They looked like they'd gone down to hell and back, but they were all smiling. We helped them out from under their packs, and they sprawled here and there against rocks to recover and eat. About an hour later, the final bunch returned from the summit to another hero's welcome. They were allowed to rest for another hour. Then we had to pack up and clear out of Camp Muir. The three hour descent to the parking lot was a lark. At least it was for someone who'd gotten a good night's rest in the hut.

Back at Base Camp, Joe and I decided to celebrate our accomplishment by buying ourselves a large pizza and gorging, just the two of us, accompanied by several cold draft beers. We ordered the pizza and two beers, which came to the whopping sum of $30.00. While waiting for our order, we joined our guides, Jon, Win, and the others, at a picnic table, where they were to preside over a formal end to the climb by handing out certificates and handshakes to all participants. We'd planned to attend the formalities and then move on to our pizza and beer. It took so long for our group to gather around the guides that the waiter delivered our pizza just as the gathering had gotten underway. He'd done a head count and thoughtfully brought along eight plates. He set it down in the middle of the table. Joe and I glanced at each other in alarm.

"Need anything else?" the waiter asked me.

"No! You've done more than enough."

Within seconds, the pizza had been divided up among the first eight people to grab, which, fortunately, included Joe and me. Joe managed to snag two.

Then There Is No Mountain

I was handed a Participant Certificate by Jon. He shook my hand, which meant and means much more to me than the certificate, considering his elite status as one who's successfully climbed Mount Everest. After we'd all raised our glasses to each other, Jon told us his Everest story. An email list was passed around. Then we all drifted apart, to prepare for the return to our separate lives. My first act of preparation was to go back to the café counter and order a cheeseburger, and another beer. Joe and I packed and loaded the Land Rover. Then we soaked for a few minutes in the Whitaker Bunkhouse's outdoor hot tub, not saying much, as the light grew soft.

Seattle

The mountain paced us on our right, shining white, and awesome in its enormity. "We were up there!" we kept shouting to each other. "Way the hell up *there!*" We were back in the Rover, rolling north to Seattle.

It was a challenging day to be visiting Seattle, especially without knowing its streets. There was extensive street work going on, causing us to resort to several of our well-practiced U-turns. Also a charity marathon of some sort was ongoing, which resulted in its own set of barricades. Finally, we parked in a pay lot about a mile and a half south of the city center, and set out on an urban hike. We immediately felt better once we were out of the Rover and navigating on our feet.

I'd told Joe about an art gallery I'd seen in Pioneer Square nearly twenty years before, which seemed to have built up its business by acquiring an original Edward S. Curtiss folio, dismantling it, matting and framing each of the prints separately, and offering them for enormous sums. I'd been scandalized at the time that anyone could be crass enough to destroy one of those sacred works, and then expect to be rewarded for it. I'd assumed that the gallery would be long gone by now, the owner having fled the country to live a life of ease in the tropics from his ill-gotten gains, but there it was, still. Joe and I stepped inside. The proprietors had diversified their stock, compared to my memory, but several Curtiss prints still hung on the wall for sale. Grave, dark eyes gazed steadily back at us as we examined them. We assumed the skeptical attitudes of men seriously considering a purchase or two, which had the desired effect of keeping the salesperson at bay, so as not to disturb the delicate equilibrium of our weighty decision-making process.

Those beautiful faces haunted me (they haunt me still) as we hiked up to the Pike Place Market to join the mad crush of *hoi polloi*. We stopped in Elliott Bay Book Company and relaxed for a while over a crossword and coffee. We rambled the avenues for a while, catching glimpses of Puget Sound and the islands, and just feeling for the life of the city.

Eventually, we made our way south to the Rover. We drove down to the town of SeaTac, checked in to a Motel 6 near the airport, and had supper at a diner improbably named Route 66. This name had a special resonance for me, since I'd once owned a likewise-named diner in Tulsa, actually on Route 66. The significance of this was lost on our waitress.

Later, while lying in bed waiting for sleep, I opened the Gideon's Bible and read from the book of Kings: *"Now King David was old, advanced in years; and they put covers on him, but he could not get warm. Therefore his servants said to him, "Let a young woman, a virgin, be sought for our lord the king, and let her stand before the king, and let her care for him; and let her lie in his bosom, that our lord the king may be warm." So they sought for a lovely young woman throughout all the territory of Israel, and found Abishag the Shunammite, and brought her to the king. The young woman was very lovely; and she cared for the king, and served him; but the king did not know her...."* I closed the bible, remembering when I'd first woke up from surgery the year before, a seedless husk, bone cold, and how I'd quaked so uncontrollably, under heavy blankets, until I'd passed back out. Then I remembered how the cold had again crept into me while I'd sat in the cloud on the side of Mount Rainier, struggling for breath, wondering where my strength had gone. I remembered, too, how I'd struggled to stand again, there on the mountainside. One day, like my father before me, I'll stand for the last time, not knowing, as I walk about my business, that my feet will never bear my weight again.

There's never a reason to linger in a Motel 6, so we were up and rolling south on I-5 nice and early. At Olympia we headed west to eventually make our way to Highway 101 South. As we drove past Satsop, Joe became excited at the unmistakable sight of nuclear power plant cooling towers, and snapped a couple of blurry pictures as we sped past. The Satsop project was never finished, and is now rumored to be trying for a second life as an office park, of all things. Joe was once a radical environmentalist, a member of Earth First, and a frontline participant in the successful uprising against the Black Fox Nuclear Power Plant project in eastern Oklahoma in the 1970s. He

120

has a bumper sticker on his decrepit farm pickup that says "Visualize Industrial Collapse," which is the radical environmentalist's answer to the bumper sticker slogan, "Visualize World Peace." Industrial collapse is exactly what you are visualizing when you look at his old Dodge pickup with its missing windows, gouged paint, dents, cracked mirrors, rusting bed, and dry-rotting tires.

Our goal was the mouth of the Columbia River. Joe is a lifelong admirer of Lewis and Clark, particularly Clark. We were going to the place where Lewis and Clark had camped and viewed the Pacific Ocean for the first time. The place where Lewis (or was it Clark?) had written *"Ocian in view. O! the joy!"* in his journal. When we got to Long Beach, Washington, Joe, like his hero Clark, would be viewing the Pacific *Ocian* for the first time.

A short distance north of the small town of Seaview, on Highway 103, we turned left, drove a block, and parked. The *ocian* was not yet in view. It writhed just beyond the small dunes a couple of hundred yards ahead between us. We sat on the tailgate and ate sandwiches made from a hunk of summer sausage and cheddar cheese left over from my climbing provisions, rough-slicing the meat and cheese with a large pocket knife. On the walk to the beach, we walked past a tiny, temporary amusement park with a miniature ferris wheel, a pony ride, and a sno-cone stand. The only customer was a boy, about five, riding one of the ponies. His parents paced nervously alongside, and the girl in the sno-cone booth leaned out her window to watch. Where the sidewalk ended, a couple of nearly empty hotels sat stubbornly facing the deserted beach.

When Joe first saw the blue-gray wind-whipped water, he didn't smile. He stared at it and walked toward it in a straight line, until he was standing in it. "O! The joy!" He shouted over the roaring wind and thundering waves. I took his picture. The noise level of water and wind made it a chore to converse, so we barely spoke as we walked along the mostly deserted beach, separately and together. The wind was intense. It blew hard, maybe 25 or 30 m.p.h., nonstop and from the north, straight down the beach, so that above the dryline everything was being sandblasted and buried in the blowing sand. We saw three women walking around looking for a place to spread their blankets in the sand for an afternoon at the beach. They were wrapped head to toe in their blankets, carrying baskets, and looking like robed and burka'd refugees as they veered aimlessly in the wind. Joe and I walked around for nearly an hour, just experiencing the strangeness of the place. We walked past a couple lying entwined in the sand, their heads and upper torsos hidden beneath the upper fold of their blanket which was pinned down over them by the relentless wind. They lay as still as driftwood. The sand was beginning to drift up against their blanketed heads.

We made our way through the low dunes to a boardwalk, which we took back toward the streetmouth. When we got off the boardwalk, I saw a lone figure looking out the glass wall of a bar on the top floor of a four-story hotel. I supposed him to be the world's loneliest bartender, looking out beyond the hotel's empty parking lot to the northern horizon.

We drove south to the famous Lewis and Clark campsite, parked in the small roadside parking area, and took our pictures in front of the big sign. A few miles later, we crossed the Columbia River to Astoria, Oregon, a small port city pleasantly situated along the bluffs where the river empties into the estuary and its waters mix with the sea. South along Highway 101 past Seaside, we turned onto Highway 26 and angled across Oregon's low coastal range to Portland.

When we arrived at Nicole and Lisa's, Louise and I gave each other long hugs and kisses. "Oh, it's nice to see you," I whispered. It felt as if I'd been gone from her longer than five days. Nicole and Lisa fed us well, and it was good to be in back in their sweet, airy, familiar home. We spent a pleasant evening with Joe and me telling Louise, Nicole, Lisa, the dog and the two cats all about our adventures on the mountain and the people we'd met there. When I became drowsy, I broke away before the rest, wished everyone a good night, took a hot bath and went to bed. Within a few minutes, Louise slipped in beside me. We lay close in the dark and spoke very quietly until we fell asleep against each other.

Portland

I woke up early, made coffee, padded through the dark, quiet house, and took a cup out onto their deck. The crescent moon hung low in the eastern sky like a tensed bow. I followed the line of an imaginary arrow fired from the bow of the moon, and realized it would continue below the horizon on a flight straight to the center of the sun, every time, without fail. A few minutes later, the buoyant sun cleared the horizon just where the imaginary arrow had predicted, and all heaven broke loose.

The next two days were free-form relaxation. We took walks separately and together in the neighborhood, under warm, sunny skies. We lounged around the house flipping through magazines and newspapers, sipping coffee, and engaging in desultory conversations, the threads of which we dropped and picked back up in random ways at random times, or not at all.

Portland is a city of neighborhoods, each one a self-contained district with its own character. Nicole and Lisa's neighborhood, called Multnomah Village, is a concentration of locally owned cafes, boutiques, antique stores, taverns, galleries, a grocery store, a bank, and a toy store. Louise and I shopped in the toy store for presents for our two-year old grandson, Braydon. We got him a toy airplane, a kaleidoscope, some wooden ABC blocks and a few other toys, none of which required any form of electricity to operate. I believe a two-year-old child of today will be amused by the same things that amused a two-year-old child five centuries ago, or longer. No batteries are required to make Braydon happy. That alone would be reason enough for us to love him, but reason has nothing to do with the pangs of love Louise and I feel whenever we think of him.

Joe's wife, Laura, would be flying into Portland along with Annie, a twenty-year-old German citizen who had been Joe and Laura's foreign exchange student a couple of years before. She'd come back to see them for an

American vacation. They were to arrive at Portland International about 10:30 p.m.

In the afternoon, Louise and I took a city bus downtown to visit the Portland Art Museum, which has at least one of just about everything, including a Van Gogh of which I'd never even seen a reproduction in Louise's large library of art books. Everything I know about art (such as I do), I've learned from her. I've absorbed from her an orderly vision of the Grand Continuum of Art, unfurling through the centuries like brightly colored ribbons. That, however, tells me nothing about the mysterious magic that happens when Louise herself puts paint on canvas. I once thought I'd come to understand her alchemy in time, but I was wrong. How she does what she does has only become more mysterious.

She paints in oils. Her palette is a bouquet of every color under the sun. If you stand up close to one of her paintings, the paint itself becomes a sensual treat for the eyes, a marvelous chaos of delicious colors. Step back and all that marvelous chaos coalesces into a harmonious image spun from the world around us. Louise will use a dozen colors or more to paint a white vase, and what you see is unquestionably an image of *that* vase, *that* white. The image is usually more beautiful than the object itself. How does she do it? I'll never know.

Walking through an art museum with Louise is a complex experience. Her deep, passion-driven knowledge of art history makes her the best guide imaginable—an ideal, personal docent. On the other hand, Louise has such a personal identification with the renowned artists of the European tradition that she likes to linger among their works, and her passions can be obscure to those less schooled. We work art galleries at different paces, so, inevitably, we drift apart. I move on, to check back in with her every few minutes. We also have different interests. She lingered for quite a while in front of Courbet's self-portrait in the Portland Art Museum. They also happened to be showing an exhibition of the works of M. C. Escher, which I was keen to see. Louise declined to sully her higher-plane experience with a visit to that gallery, preferring instead to return Courbet's smoldering gaze. After the museum we strolled through a park, and caught a bus back to Multnomah Village.

Later, Nicole and Lisa took Joe, Louise, and me to a barbeque place they knew of across the river. When our food arrived, I raised my beer glass and said, a bit formally, but from the heart: "Nicole and Lisa, your generosity, and your hospitality, has meant so much to us. Although we'd welcome the opportunity, I don't know how we could ever really repay you. It seems all we can do for now is thank you." I looked into Nicole's eyes. "Thank you," I said. She blushed beautifully.

We'd driven two vehicles to dinner, so the women went back to Nicole and Lisa's, and Joe and I took the Rover downtown to kill some time before picking up Laura & Annie at the airport. We went to Powell's Books and quickly separated, each to our own explorations. Mine soon took me back out onto the street. I'd lived in Portland for a few months in 1978. I'd stayed in a seedy downtown hotel (whose name was long ago lost to me), and I wanted to find it. I'd remembered it being near Powell's. I walked down an avenue, studying the buildings, and within a couple of blocks, I recognized it. It was still a hotel, but it had gone "boutique." The old street level lobby, where I had slipped past the sharp-eyed desk clerks on a few occasions to avoid the subject of weekly rent, had become an upscale restaurant. From the sidewalk I looked up at the third-floor window that I guessed must have been my old room, and I remembered a moment I'd once had looking out that window. An old chill settled over me.

I'd drifted out to Portland with a friend in the summer of 1978. We'd first gone to the suburbs to look up an old army buddy of his. We'd slept on the couches and floors of his buddy and his buddy's friends for a while, but I'd never gotten along with any of them. As soon as I found a job through a temp agency, I moved to this downtown flophouse. I worked day-labor jobs for minimum wage, confronting every day this simple rule of economics: if, daily, you make a little less than it takes for food, rent, transportation, and the like, then every day is a day closer to the final zero sum. That's the day you find the door to your room locked, with all your things still inside, and you have no ideas for your next meal or bed. I was doing the math in my room, one evening after work, when I sat by the window to look down for a while at the cheerful streetlife gathering in the twilight. My eyes drifted up and I saw directly across the street from me an old man, framed in his window as I was in mine. I could see him clearly in the low, slanting sunlight. He was unshaven, he had bags under his eyes, and his gray hair was combed only with his fingers. He was looking steadily at me. I felt a chill in my soul. For a moment, I couldn't look away, but then I jumped up and backed away from the window and closed the drapes. I stood in the dark, my heart racing. I'd seen myself in that window across the street, looking back at me through the shabby years of a wasted life. I had to change my drifting ways. I had to make some connections. I had to find some friends. I needed a lover, an apartment, a car, a stable job. I had to get with the program.

As I stood there, years later, looking up at my old window, I remembered another strange encounter I'd had, back in those old days. This was an encounter with a woman. I'd taken a booth in a café around the corner from the hotel and ordered a sandwich and a Coke. A wan woman sat alone in the booth before me, watching me, holding my eyes when I glanced up. On the plate before her was a half-eaten sandwich. When I glanced up again, she was still looking at me and again didn't look away. I nodded and said hello. She and her sandwich were in my booth in an instant.

"Hi," she breathed, and tossed off her name as if it meant nothing. "What's yours?" she asked, and waited with wide-eyed impatience, as if it meant everything. I told her my name.

Within moments, it seemed, and after only a few words, words that I could never remember later, she'd become dependent on me. I'd agreed to tap into my week's bus fare and pay for her sandwich, along with my own. I also bought us each a cup of coffee and a piece of pie. She ate quietly, economically, and with a focus that excluded myself. She wasn't much for small talk. She had no money, she told me, but she had to eat. Her teeth were small and even. Her wrists were as thin as broom handles, her hair lank. When it was time to go, she asked, softly, "Do you live around here?"

"I have a room around the corner."

"I'd like to see it."

We went to my room, slipping discreetly past the desk clerk (because my weekly rent was a day late and going to get later). She was so thin I had to probe with my fingers to find her, inside her clothes, as I undressed her. Her skin was cool. When I made love to her, she held onto me, light as a bird, and was nearly silent except for her quick breaths. Afterward, she flew. I never saw her again. I was never sure if she was trading sex for food, or was simply hungry for both. The way it played out, the whole scenario was open for interpretation.

I'd soon gotten a job in a hospital as a clerk in the radiology department, shuffling files. Nothing was digitized in those days, of course, so there were vast storerooms filled with thick patient files. Down among those storerooms, I'd made friends among my coworkers, had a couple of flings among the pretty women there, and after a time, had saved enough money to move into an apartment. In short, I'd begun to change my drifter ways. Then I got a message from home.

My father had had an aneurism, was in a coma, and wasn't expected to live. By the end of the next day, I was on my way back to Indiana. I remembered all that, and more, as I stood on the sidewalk looking up at my old window.

As I made my way back to Powell's to find Joe, the streets had filled with people. Folks were out for a summer's night on the town, and I remembered one more incident from my old Portland days. It had been somewhere along that same street, and the street had been similarly full of people out and about. I was with a couple whom I'd recently met, and as we strolled together arm in arm from one bar to another, I spied a young woman as she stepped out onto a second-floor fire escape landing. My tongue loosened by alcohol, and by the generally upbeat vibe of the street, I stopped on the sidewalk and called up to her, "What light through yonder window breaks? It is the east, and Juliet is the sun!" "O Romeo, Romeo, wherefore art thou, Romeo?" she called back down, laughingly. We then spontaneously improvised a slapdash version of the balcony scene as a crowd gathered around me and, led by my companions, cheered us on. When it began to fall apart after a few lines, I bowed deeply, and bid her adieu. We blew each other kisses, and I and my friends moved on.

I used to obsess over the random nature of memory. The events that you might consider pivotal, precious, or terrible in your life story seem no more likely to be retained than other events of no identifiable meaning. I remember being momentarily overcome with loneliness as I looked down our family's sloping lawn in the flat, gray twilight when, I was 3 or 4. I remember a winter sun rising into a pink-smudged sky through the black claws of a distant copse of bare trees, when I was ten. I remember a red teapot resting on a stove in someone's kitchen, I don't know when or where. I remember my wife absent-mindedly sorting through the mail one afternoon, when I was fifty. I remember hearing Hank Williams from a distant, tinny radio, but where was I, and when was it? I remember my father ordering a cup of black coffee in a diner, when I was eighteen. I'd seen him order coffee in that diner countless times, but for some reason I remember that one. But I don't remember the first time I drove a car, or kissed a girl. I don't remember my high school graduation. Why don't I remember those things?

You and I have forgotten almost everything that has ever happened to us. How much of our lives do we remember? Less than one percent? How can we be sure of anything, once we realize that? I used to try to force myself to remember certain things as they were occurring, because they were too meaningful, or just too sweet, too to be allowed to slip away. *Remember this! Pay attention, now—smell it! Hear it! Take this all in. Commit it to memory.* I would make a point of recalling such incidents afterwards, rolling the sensations, the emotions, over in my mind, savoring them. But those incidents were no more likely to remain in memory than anything else.

Meanwhile, back in the summer of 2009, in Portland, Oregon, I was on my way to rejoin Joe at Powell's Bookstore. After I found him, we took a wayward route back to the Rover so I could show him my old digs. Then we headed out to the airport to pick up Laura.

The long oval approach to the Portland Airport is similar in its grand scale and dimensions to what I imagine the approach to the palace at Versailles might be like. When we got to the parking garage, with its neon signs and arrows directing us off the oval and into its maw, Joe mistakenly drove right past it. As a result, we executed a U-turn on a grand scale. Like pilots practicing a touch-and-go landing, we slowed as we approached the main terminal, and then accelerated away from it, in a big arc, until we eventually reached the other end of the Great Oval, far from the terminal, and lined up for our second approach. This time, working as closely as a pilot and co-pilot, we managed to successfully catch the ramp into the garage and park.

Laura and Annie's flight was one-and-a-half hours late. We filled the time reading, people-watching, and finally sitting and staring at the spot where we expected them to emerge. It was past midnight when they finally walked up to us. It would have been past 2:00 a.m. in Tulsa, where Laura had just come from. It would have been God-knows-what-time in Germany, where Annie had started out a couple of days before. They were tired. I hung back so Joe could give his women good, welcoming hugs.

We made it back to Nicole and Lisa's with a minimum of fuss and, if I remember correctly, no U-turns, although that seems unlikely. It was so late when we arrived that there was only a brief, whispered introduction to our hosts, some quick instructions regarding the bathroom and other practicalities, and then everyone dispersed to beds. In the morning, Joe, Laura, Annie, and I would begin our roadtrip back to Tulsa after breakfast.

The Redwood Country

When morning came, and everyone got up and organized, Nicole and Lisa wanted us all to eat a farewell breakfast at the Original Pancake House down the road from their house. "This is the *original* original," Lisa wanted us to know.

The place was an immaculate, flawless setting right out of the 1950s. There was a reasonably short wait for a table. The food was spectacular. We all ate with great gusto, guzzling coffee and orange juice, shouting happily over the din, as if we'd won something, putting away waffles, pancakes, blintzes, omelets, and muffins. Laura generously paid for everyone, which caused me to breathe a sigh of relief. Nicole and Lisa had sheltered and fed Joe and me for four nights, and sheltered Laura and Annie for one. Joe, who operates on a cash-only basis at all times, had run out of cash days before while we were still at Rainier Base Camp, because he'd been covering many of my expenses. I had then covered Joe and myself on our jaunt up to Seattle and out to the coast, which had left me and Louise very low on funds, which I had further depleted by picking up the tab at the barbeque joint the night before.

Back at Nicole and Lisa's, we packed the Land Rover, and everyone congregated in the driveway for hugs, thanks, and farewells. Louise and I gave ourselves a few private moments for a quiet goodbye. She'd be flying back to Tulsa in two days, and I was scheduled to arrive there in six. Joe and I had driven out to Portland with my wife, and would now be driving back with his, who, along with Annie, would be getting off at Albuquerque and spending a couple of days in Santa Fe with a friend. They planned to attend the opera there.

As soon as we got to the highway, we made a wrong turn. Our intended route ran south out of town on I-5 but we found ourselves driving north instead, all the way downtown. Joe was driving, and Laura was sitting in the co-pilot's seat. They engaged in some spirited navigational debate along the way. We all agreed we had to turn around, but how, and where? When an opportunity arose, Joe exited the highway onto a city street, entered an office parking lot through the exit, and exited via the entrance. This got us headed back south on a street parallel to I-5. Eventually, we found an entrance ramp onto I-5 southbound and headed out of Portland.

The Willamette Valley is a broad, north-south valley, with the Cascades to the east, and the Coast Range to the west. Beyond the Cascades, the land opens out into the endless, arid Basin and Range provinces of the American West. Beyond the Coast Range is the Pacific Ocean. In between them, the Willamette River, running north to the Columbia, long ago wallowed out this green, fertile, idyllic valley. We drove through hay meadows, horse farms, vineyards, berry farms, and farm towns.

At Grant's Pass, where the Cascades and the Coast Ranges squeeze closer together, we stopped to stretch and have a light lunch in a local coffee shop. Grant's Pass reminded me of Tahlequah, Oklahoma. In both towns, the local businesses are more oriented toward serving the local residents' needs than those of tourists. The Rogue River flows by Grant's Pass, like the Illinois River flows by Tahlequah. The low, rugged, wooded hills of the Coast Range are not unlike the Ozarks, if you squint. The muddy pickups parked at the tire store, the hardware store, the coffee shop, and the canoe rental place -and the plain-faced, plain-dressed, well-booted families on the sidewalks- made me say to Laura: "These people are hillbillies." I meant that as a compliment. I come from a long, proud line of hillbilly stock. Laura considered my remark for a couple of moments with an inscrutable look, and decided not to reply. Back in the Rover, I saw on the map that, coincidentally, a few miles south of town, they even had their own Illinois River. I wanted this to prove something, but it didn't, so I didn't bring it up.

We exited I-5 at Grant's Pass, on to U.S. Highway 199, which angled us southwest toward the coast. It wasn't long before we spotted the first redwoods, spiking up above the canopy along ridge lines. By the time we crossed into California, the forest was thick with redwoods. At Crescent City, we turned on to Highway 101, the Coast Highway. Once we were deep in the giant redwoods we stopped at a pullout, got out of the vehicle and stood there for a few moments just gawking, like everyone else who's ever been there. A loop trail beckoned us irresistibly into the woods. With every step into the woods our communion with the trees' strange majesty became less shared and more solitary. Within a few steps, we'd drifted apart from each other, and we walked in silence, each at our own pace. I glided down the path, slow and steady through the deep stillness, in a state of high awareness. I heard the muted chimes of birds passing secret signals to each other, far above. The slanted light, filtered through three hundred feet of canopy, settled tenderly over the profusion of ferns crowding the floor. These ferns were as tall as we were. They, almost as much as the trees, served to shrink us to our true dimensions. Tiny creatures we were, able to hide within, maybe even live within, the shadowed folds of the trees' buttressing roots. The treetops were a world away, too far for us to see, maybe stirring in breezes we couldn't feel, under a blue sky we couldn't see. After a few turns in the path, I'd lost sight of Annie, Joe, and Laura. Each, I assumed, was walking along in their own private reverie. After a few more turns, I stopped to allow them to catch up. Annie arrived first, and we spoke in whispers, not wanting to wake ourselves from our strange dream. When Joe and Laura arrived, their eyes filled with the soft light of the place, we all walked through the dreamscape together.

After several minutes, Joe realized that none of us had really looked at the board with the trail map. We'd glanced at it, and seen that it was a loop trail, but none of us had checked the scale. Was it a half-mile loop or a ten-mile loop? We stopped to discuss it. Joe thought we should turn around. I agreed. Turning back was a known route of known distance. It was getting late in the day. Laura, who'd been leading the way, seemed to take this personally. She knew, she said, that the Rover was just ahead. Joe, with a show of patience, replied to her that she couldn't know that. Laura replied, with a show of impatience, that it would be pointless, and *further*, to turn back. Anna and I looked off into the ferns. Laura's voice began to rise, and Joe's began to lower, as each dug into position. Laura announced that she would go on alone, and we could do what we liked. Joe informed her that he couldn't allow her to do that. I mumbled my agreement with Joe. Eventually, Laura gave in and headed back down the trail, leading the way, but making it clear that she was not happy about it. Joe glanced at me with relief and rushed ahead to catch up with her. Anna and I lagged behind. We threaded our way back among the head-high ferns, along a sun-dappled stream, through tunnels of deep shadow, and around thirty-foot-diameter tree trunks with cathedral-scale buttresses. When we caught up with Laura and Joe, they were at peace, waiting for us. We retraced our steps back to the Rover, got back on the road, and continued south. Laura massaged Joe's neck while he drove. Annie looked out the window.

The shabby towns along the Coast Highway, with their weeds, rust, and closed businesses, are not unlike certain Oklahoma small towns that seem to have outlived their usefulness. By the time we got to Arcata, it was dark and the evening fog had thickened. We began to watch for a motel. Ah, a Best Western sign up ahead! Joe took the next exit. We needed to make a left turn at the top of the ramp, then cross over the highway to get to the motel. At the top of the ramp we confronted the novelty of a small traffic circle, instead of the usual simple stop sign. This creative California traffic engineering required us to go three-fourths of the way around the circle to make our left. Joe only made it half-way around before he exited the circle— despite Laura and me calling out, "No!" "Wait!" It was too late. We were on the entrance ramp back onto the highway. "What just happened?" Joe wondered aloud.

We'd have to continue south to the next exit, take it, cross over, and backtrack north to the motel exit. What followed was our most elaborate, largest scale U-turn yet, a fleur-de-lis flourish on the line of our passage. Laura and I, leaning forward in our seats, talked Joe onto the next exit ramp, which looped us back up and over the highway. Unfortunately, there was no traffic circle on the other side to loop us back onto the northbound ramp. In fact, there was a median preventing us from making the necessary left turn. We were driving east on an unknown divided road, through a night fog. We were tired and getting further every moment from the highway, and from the Best Western. After a couple of miles with no place to turn around, Joe suddenly slowed and swerved left into the center median ditch. The rest of us could only hang on as we bounced down and up the other side, and onto the pavement. Soon we were back on the Coast Highway headed north. I saw Annie grinning at the craziness of it all. We exited by the big, warm, bright Best Western sign. At the top of the ramp was another dreaded traffic circle.

We just had to make it one-quarter of the way around the circle, exit right, and we'd be on the way to crisp, clean sheets and a good night's rest. Once in the circle, Joe pretended to be missing our turn, causing us all to yell at him. Just kidding. In a few minutes, we were unpacking into a spacious suite. The ladies took the bedroom, and Joe and I each opened up a sofabed in the living room. Soon we turned out the lights, and the day was done.

Without fuss, soon after rising, we were rolling south, fast-food breakfasts and Starbucks coffees in hand. By the time we got to Humboldt State Park and the Avenue of the Giants, the morning fog had dissipated to reveal a mild, sunny morning. We pulled into a parking lot at a trailhead after threading our way through the giant trees along the avenue for a few miles. We were pretty much the only ones there. The air was soft and calm. The morning light slanted dramatically down through the redwoods. This time we studied the map together at the trailhead and then set out for a short walk on the loop trail. I was eager for a workout, so I quickly left Joe, Laura, and Annie behind as my legs devoured the winding path in big gulps. The woods was as still as a photograph. When I got back to the trailhead, I stood still for a couple of minutes until my breathing calmed and a wave of euphoria washed over me. The near-silence of the woods was full enough to drown out the sounds of my own thoughts. I set out for a second lap, released from self-awareness, gliding in silence at a natural pace, riding a rolling wave of *now*. I felt the slight temperature differences as I passed from shadow to light. I drank in shifting combinations of subtle aromas. I was weightless, my body had evaporated into the world, and only my senses remained. I eddied around each bend in the dappled path without will, without goal, and with no sense of time.

When I arrived again at the trailhead, I realized that I had expected to catch up to the others as they strolled along, but hadn't. I walked over to the parking lot and found Joe and Annie. Laura was missing. Joe had expected her to come out with me. I walked back over to the trailhead and set out on the trail starting at the end, instead of the beginning. After backtracking a short distance I encountered her, happily making her way along. She'd taken a second loop off the first loop, presumably for a few minutes of solitude and a bit more exercise. When we got back to the parking lot, Joe's relief overcame his agitation, so he didn't fuss.

Mendocino

We exited Highway 101 at Leggett, onto State Highway 1, to cut over to Mendocino. This curvy stretch of two-lane road became the perfect platform for Joe to exhibit his skills in the art and practice of the U-turn. It seemed, in fact, that he'd been preparing for this ever since Tulsa, honing his skills. The next 40 miles was a continuous series of back-to-back U-turns, hairpins, cliffhangers, and sidewinders, all of which Joe negotiated with the nonchalance of a master in top form. He kept the Rover at the maximum speed possible, without causing anyone to spill their drinks, or grab for handholds. He steered with one finger through one-eighties, while conversationally riffing with me on great men of history, from Thucydides to Muir to Churchill, using the rearview mirror for eye contact. He squeaked us past logging trucks coming the other way without seeming to notice them. Thickly forested canyons with sheer walls waited to receive us, only a battered guardrail away. When we finally got to the coast, we all got out and stood on the rim of a low sea-cliff and watched the waves until the world stopped spinning inside our heads. It was a lonely spot, and no one said much as we stood there looking out.

Mendocino is an isolated, small coastal town. Joe parked the Rover facing downhill on Lansing Street. We strolled a few blocks, stopping to ponder the mysterious sculpture atop the cupola of the Masonic Hall. An Angel of Death braids a young woman's hair. The woman is doing something with a book laid atop a broken pillar. An hourglass stands at her feet. What the hell?

Just like tourists can be easy to spot, so can locals. The locals all had the same rough, weathered look: lean, with deeply lined faces and washed out eyes. They looked like desert people, but this coastal terrain was lush and damp. After having lunch in a boisterous tavern, we got coffees to go at a coffee stand, climbed into the Rover, buckled up, and took off. Joe pulled into a service station two blocks later, at the bottom of the hill. I assumed for fuel, but I was wrong.

"Something's not right," Joe announced.

"What?"

"Transmission. It won't go into gear."

"What?"

"I hit the gas, it just revs up. It's slipping. We need to check the fluid level." He jumped out, raised the hood, and disappeared behind it. I joined him after a couple of minutes. We shared a common American middle-aged man's frustration: we'd grown up tinkering with cars, and knew our way around under the hoods of cars we'd grown up with, but over time, what we'd found under the hoods of our cars resembled more and more a black box, and less and less an engine. The Land Rover was the ultimate example. Nothing in the engine compartment made sense to us. They might as well have put a sticker on the hood: *"No user-serviceable parts inside."* We couldn't even find the transmission dipstick. We dug the owner's manual out of the glove box and searched for some reference to adding transmission fluid. Then we saw: *"Transmission fluid is factory-filled in a sealed system for the life of the vehicle."*

Joe's face had the clamped jaw and neutral expression of a man concealing a bomb of panic. I suppose mine was the same. The next few minutes were difficult. We were stranded in an isolated small town with no chance of anyone local being able to diagnose, let alone repair, the Land Rover. Since it wasn't a fluid leak—we searched for signs of leakage and found none—we could only conclude that it was something worse. The transmission itself had evidently failed. The Rover sat there, blocking the service station's gas pumps, immovable as a boulder. It was suggested that we give it another try. Joe had fallen deep into crisis mode. He replied that there was no point in trying it again. After all, nothing had changed. He didn't want to cause worse damage. He began leafing through the manual for a toll-free number. He asked the station attendant where the closest Land Rover dealership was. She shrugged, but then went to look it up for us. It was again suggested that we test it. Joe didn't reply. Well, what did we have to lose? *Come on, let's try it and see what happens.* To prove the pointlessness, and to stop us from annoying him while he tried to think, Joe sat in the driver's seat, turned it on, and put it into gear. To everyone's surprise, and relief, we pulled smoothly out of the service station lot and onto the street, just as the station attendant came hustling out with a phonebook in her hand. We accelerated up the hill, everyone alert for any hint of a problem. It seemed to be fine.

"Okay," Joe said as we passed the city limit sign. "I just figured it out."

"What?"

"Everything's okay. Nothing's wrong."

"What happened?"

"I had my wallet sitting on the shifter console, and it blocked the shifter from going into gear. When I felt it hit the edge of my wallet, it felt like it does when it hits its slot for drive, but the transmission was still in neutral. My fault. We're okay."

We were all so relieved, and so glad to see Joe's relief, that we couldn't even give him a hard time about it. It could have happened to any of us.

"Hell," I said, "that's probably how all the locals have ended up here. I bet we could've made a go of it. Turn this Land Rover into a taco stand, work the tourist trade."

"Help out with the marijuana harvest. Dance at the harvest festival."

"Marry Annie here off into a local family." (Annie rolled her eyes.)

"Join the local Masons."

"Too bad we're gonna miss all that," I sighed. Mendocino receded in our rearview mirrors.

We made our way back over the coast range to Highway 101 and headed south through the endless beauty of California's wine country. We'd hoped to mosey along, stopping at a few wineries along the way, but, as the man said, we had reservations to keep, and miles to go before we could sleep, or words to that effect, so we kept on the move. At Santa Rosa I took the wheel and drove us into the Bay Area megalopolis of Petaluma, Novato, San Rafael, Sausalito, and finally, the Golden Gate Bridge, that beautiful red gateway to the mystical white city of San Francisco.

San Francisco

I'd wanted to visit San Francisco all my life. My parents had moved to Vallejo, across the bay, in the spring of 1951 with my two-year-old big brother, Danny. By the time they caught a train back to Arkansas in February, 1952, my mother was seven months pregnant with me. I've always had a romantic vision of the San Francisco my parents saw when they were in the area, not long after World War II. I saw sailors and soldiers in gangs on the streets, and girls in old-fashioned hairdos. I imagined big band, bebop, fog, and fedoras, and ships lit up in the harbor at night, and Kerouac and Ginsberg bounding along the streets, talking a mile a minute.

In Vallejo, my father went to work as a mechanic for my mother's great uncle, at his service station. They never really got along with him, the story goes, so in early '52, they took the train back to Arkansas. My father was made miserably seasick by the rocking train, the whole trip. For the rest of his life, he couldn't ride in the backseat of any car, claiming carsickness. My mother, age 21, had an incapacitated husband, a crying three-year-old, and me churning around in her belly as they chugged and rocked over the Sierra Nevadas, across deserts, and, days later, back into the humid arms of Dixie, where they found work in the timber camps. They both worked, turning pine trees into telephone poles, outside Warren, Arkansas, not far from the Louisiana border. I was born there in April. Six weeks later, we all moved to Indiana. They never did pay the hospital for delivering me. I assume the statute of limitations has now run out. This was postwar America, and the great industrial North was booming like never before (or since). My mother's sister and her husband had already gone north. Their letters described a paradise of good union factory jobs, ripe for picking, in every smoky town. We moved to Richmond, Indiana, a small industrial city set among bountiful fields with deep, rich topsoil. Sure enough, Dad found a union job in a school bus factory and the two of them raised five children there. In moving from the played-out rural South to the booming postwar industrial North, we were part of a surprisingly unacknowledged mass migration that surely rivaled or perhaps even exceeded the famous Dust Bowl migration westward.

Laura had booked us two rooms for two nights at the Intercontinental Mark Hopkins Hotel. Once we cleared the bridge, Joe, Laura, and I put into action our careful plan for navigating the twisting streets of an unfamiliar city. Utilizing our atlas, our Google Map printouts, and our in-dash GPS display panel, Laura called out the pre-planned turns to me several blocks in advance. Through no fault of hers, we'd soon entangled ourselves in a maze of one-way streets, unexpected dead-ends, and forced turns in wrong directions. But we stayed focused, and for every deviation from our plan forced upon us by the actual real world, we nimbly improvised an alternative route. Our planned frontal assault on Nob Hill thus became a probing operation. Nob Hill is a steep-sided butte running east-west. Along its spine runs California Street. The one-way streets intersecting California climb up one steep side and descend down the other. The Mark Hopkins perches at Nob Hill's eastern terminus. We caught occasional tantalizing glimpses of the hotel's tower, as we circled and probed, gradually tightening the noose. We eventually got ourselves onto California Street, approaching the hotel from the west, victory in sight.

Unfortunately, the parking entrance was not on California, but on its intersector, Mason Street, and I missed the necessary right turn. We passed the hotel, to our chagrin, and began the steep descent on the eastern end of the hill. A half-block down the steep hillside, I made an impulsive decision. "U-turn!" I yelled, and immediately spun the wheel into a sharp left turn. Laura and Annie yelped, and Joe gritted his teeth as everyone's weight was shifted to the downhill side of the turn. In retrospect, I suppose I'd risked rolling us over and down the hill, but it turned out okay. Before anyone could find something to hold on to, we were climbing back up the hill, toward the hotel. At the top I made a quick left turn, and then another into the hotel's small parking and unloading area. We were swarmed by a uniformed crew of valets, who quickly relieved us of the Land Rover and our baggage.

We were escorted into the swank lobby, where the Joe and I stood around gawking at the grand hotel splendor while Laura and Annie checked us in. We were a long way from the austere fastness of Camp Muir. Our rooms were on the fourteenth floor. Laura and Annie's room had a north view looking over the bay. Joe's and mine, across the hall, had a south-facing view of the city.

When the bellhop delivered our luggage, he asked if we had had supper. We hadn't. He recommended an Italian place a few blocks north. We all freshened up, changed clothes, and hiked down off the hill to the little bistro. There was about a 30-minute wait, and nowhere to wait except standing on the sidewalk outside, where we joined a small crowd.

Joe and Laura teased me mercilessly because I was wearing a pearl-snap shirt, an ornate Tony Lama belt, wrangler jeans, and cowboy boots. Dressing up like a cowboy on the streets of San Francisco is apparently considered funny by some people. Very funny. Funny ha-ha. Laura had ordered us some red wine to sip while we waited, and when the waitress delivered it, we toasted ourselves. "What are we drinking?" I asked Laura. "Rodney Strong," she replied. *"What? Rodney Strong?"* I asked in mock surprise. "That's my *street* name! But, please, call me Rod." And so on until we were called in to our table. The place was cramped, warm, steamy, aromatic, and noisy. Our pastas were served in large white bowls. We added ours to the laughter all around us as we enjoyed our meal. Beneath our laughter and wit, I was feeling what I can only call a deep gladness for my companions. Glad for their companionship, and glad for them as individuals.

Laura is a lawyer of the best kind—the kind who went to law school to put ideals into practice, and who hasn't forgotten that. She's spent her career as an attorney in the often-thankless trenches of public service, with Legal Aid and with the Department of the Interior. Her private practice has centered around crafting cases for little guys who've been bulldozed by big guys. She teaches aspiring lawyers to do the same at the University of Tulsa. She's also multilingual, with a natural gift for languages. At the time of our trip together, she was working on a degree in linguistics, which seems like a natural fit for a lawyer, since the law is about, as much as anything, the precise application and interpretation of language to the goings-on among people.

Then There Is No Mountain

Joe is an idealist with anarchic tendencies who would prefer not to suffer fools, but there are just too many of them besieging him on all fronts, especially the political ones. So suffer them he must, usually with gruff good humor. He's the kind of citizen we need more of: a gun-totin', amendment-quotin', plain-speakin', redneckin', squinty-eyed, wool-dyed *liberal*. He's a passionate environmentalist who's shown the courage of his convictions with Earth First and Sierra Club. He had a tempestuous career as a middle school teacher in the Tulsa Public School system. I'm sure there was never a more passionate teacher. I've no doubt that those lucky enough to have been taught by him will never forget him. He doesn't seem to have been capable of allowing bureaucratic nonsense -or the craven calculations of administrators, or the meddlesome politics of local public schools -to get between him and his obligation to his students. He's also a student of history, with a particular interest in Thucydides and the world of ancient Greece.

Joe and Laura's home is a haven for strays, mostly dogs and cats, and there are usually about a half-dozen of each in their care. They've been known to take in human strays, too, from time to time.

They go on grand adventures together. Like the time they walked all the way across England, from sea to sea. And the time they bicycled on the Underground Railroad route into Canada. And then there are the mountains they've climbed. And now, there will be the time they went to San Francisco with young Annie and with me, when we all went out to eat in a steamy, aromatic Italian restaurant.

I looked at Annie, combing her fork through her salad. Her cheeks were flushed from the steamy air. Inscrutable. Taking everything in, and giving nothing away. On a Great American Roadtrip with people, Americans, whom she trusts. Snapping pictures, laughing at everyone's jokes, riding with us like a spirit of sweetness and youth.

I raised my glass to them all.

I almost regretted the cowboy boots I'd decided to wear to dinner, when, afterwards, we were climbing back up to the hotel. We stopped for a few moments at the top of Nob Hill to watch the city bejewelling itself for night. We were tired from a long day, and growing drowsy from the pasta, so we allowed the chilling air to nudge us on to the hotel, where we were ushered in by a courteous doorman.

Laura had booked an excursion for the four of us to tour Alcatraz. Not something I would have thought of for a must-do list during a short visit to San Francisco, but it turned out to be an interesting, even entertaining, experience. But first we had to get to Pier 33 on time for the ferry she'd booked out to the island. We set off on an urban hike from the Mark Hopkins down to Pier 33. Laura had a tri-fold brochure with a simplified San Francisco street map, so she led, holding the map out front, and we all quickly became disoriented. The map would not make sense, and Laura would not relinquish it.

After Joe had failed a couple of times to snatch the map, he tried explaining to Laura that we needed to orient the map before it would make sense. We'd been standing at different street corners, spinning slowly in circles, the map in Laura's hands spinning with us and just out of Joe's reach, and then plunging ahead with Laura's best guess. When we found ourselves standing at a dead end on the edge of a cliff facing the Coit Tower, Joe was able to convince her to let him see the map. Joe oriented the map, we backtracked to Stockton Street, took it to Bay Street, and made our way to the Embarcadero, right across from the pier.

The ferry ride was a lark. Seagulls paced us, as the beautiful city receded behind us, under white scudding clouds in a soft blue sky. The first thing you see when you disembark on the island is a big hand-lettered sign on the decaying prison wall: "INDIANS WELCOME," which struck me as a mixed message. It was a reminder that after Alcatraz was abandoned by the federal government in 1963, it was reclaimed by Native American activists in 1969, under the terms of the Treaty of Fort Laramie (1868), which specified that abandoned federal land was to be returned to the Indians. Representatives from numerous tribes occupied the island from 1969 to 1971. At first, the government laid siege to the occupied island, but eventually abandoned the siege when officials realized that the occupying Indians had, in effect, imprisoned themselves. By the time the occupation petered out, it had accomplished the goal of raising public awareness of Native American issues generally. It also resulted in other abandoned federal lands around the country being returned to the tribes. The island prison is now a national park, for some reason.

The tour at Alcatraz is a self-guided tour, like they have in museums. You wear a headset and follow the recorded instructions. It is impressively produced, with the voices of former prisoners and guards telling you stories as you are directed from cellblock to cellblock: of notorious escape attempts, riots, and murders, and of the famous bad men who were imprisoned there. Their narratives are accompanied by clanging cell doors, sirens, yelling voices, gunshots, and echoing footsteps, as appropriate to the story. We each started out at a slightly different time after being given our headsets, so we didn't reconvene until we'd each returned our headsets and emerged into the gift shop an hour or so later.

After we'd bought a few souvenirs, I decided to find a men's room before we got in line for the ferry. This required me to walk back through the prison, from one end to the other, which was a strange experience with no headset. There were hundreds of men, women, and children shuffling through the cellblocks in eerie silence, each on his own personal trajectory, all guided by voices, no one making eye contact. The only sound they made was the soft rustle of their clothes as I sidled through them–The Zombies of Alcatraz. I escaped through the front door.

After Alcatraz, and after lunch, now back onshore, Joe and Laura toured a World War II-vintage submarine at Fisherman's Wharf, while Annie and I viewed the seals that had taken up residence at Pier 39. There were dozens of them, all ages, sunning themselves side by side on several floating platforms that had been arranged for them by friendly human beings. They were, or pretend to be, indifferent to the human gawkers nearby. Now and then a new seal would pop up from under the waves and clamber aboard with the others, greeted by challenges or kisses, it was hard to tell which. Sometimes this arrival would squeeze another one off into the water, where it might play a while before climbing laboriously aboard the next platform. I took Annie's picture with them in the background. She smiled with delight.

I sometimes worried about Annie, being trapped for such a journey with three middle-aged Americans, who sometimes bickered, were sometimes confused, and who often engaged in arcane conversations for which she could have no reference points for reasons of age, culture, or language. Did she long for a couple of hours free of us? She was twenty years old, and very pretty. Did she wish to flirt with the boys whose eyes she caught? Would she have liked to make new friends among the other girls her age strolling along the Embarcadero? She never let on. I hope her memories of her time with us are good ones.

We spent the rest of the afternoon amiably hiking the hills of San Francisco. Climbing Telegraph Hill was a strenuous workout, which we enjoyed. We found ourselves in the midst of a flock of feral, crazy-talking parrots along the way. We even enjoyed getting lost as we searched for "Jack Kerouac's Love Shack"—an irresistible, and tantalizingly vague, red dot on our street map. Evidently, the current resident of said shack is not keen on having his or her home as a tourist attraction, because there isn't a plaque, sign, light, or any other indicator of which house on the short, dead-end block is the site where Kerouac wrote "On The Road." We know we saw it. We know we stood in front of it. We just don't know which house was *it*. Annie was curious about the significance of our quest, so on the way back to the Mark Hopkins, I gave her a brief history of the Beats, my thoughts on their place in twentieth-century American literature, and their influence on the later counter-culture of the Sixties. I don't have any deep knowledge or original insights about these things, but I gave her the best overview I could.

That evening, in the ebb and flow between our rooms, Laura and I happened to be alone for a couple of minutes in her room. We stood at the window looking at the bay. "Laura," I said. "I never thought I'd have this experience. To see San Francisco. To stay in a place like this. And I never would have, if you hadn't made it possible." She'd been paying for everything since she'd arrived in Portland, because Joe and I had both spent all we had, and because she could. "Thank you," I said to her reflection in the window. "You're welcome," her reflection replied.

147

Then There Is No Mountain

Laura had a vague memory of eating at a Basque restaurant on a previous visit to San Francisco, so Joe Googled around on his laptop until we came up with four possibilities. None of them was the one Laura thought she remembered but one, Iluna, at 701 Union, was within a reasonable walking distance. We viewed its menu online and agreed that it sounded interesting. When we got there, the hostess asked us, in an exotic accent, if we had a reservation. "No, we don't," I replied. She nodded slightly, and then paused for a moment before she said, "Thees way, please. Four?" We nodded enthusiastically, and she gathered four menus and led us to the best table in the room. The restaurant was on the corner of Union and Powell, and our table was in that very corner of the room, giving us ringside seats to the bustling streetlife gathering for evening. The room was at once dark and light, due to dark wood furniture countered by full length windows along both outer walls. The furniture was modern, with simple lines. The fading sunlight was augmented by warm light from hanging lamps.

Joe and Laura ordered tapas, Annie ordered a salad (she seemed to eat only salads), and I ordered a Basque chicken breast sauté with chorizo, with an appetizer of broiled plums wrapped in bacon. Everyone shared bites as we swooned through, and lingered over, the meal. For dessert I ordered Riz au Lait Orange Zest, Laura ordered Chestnut Cream Crème Brûlée, and Joe, Fondant au Chocolat Raspberry Coulis. Annie passed on dessert. Again, we all shared bites (including Annie, with only minimal urging), and each bite I took was the best bite of anything I'd ever had in my life, including the one just before. I ordered coffee and Joe ordered a glass of expensive port, to finish things off. Sated, we sipped, making desultory comments as we gazed out onto the street, and around the room, which had filled up during the course of our meal. The colorful pageant of night on the street floated past our windows. Across the street, we saw Colonel Sanders, a hippie, and a midget duck into a doorway, which looked like a good joke being acted out. They stood in the doorway and passed a joint around for a couple of minutes before stepping back out and slipping around a corner. We felt as though we'd missed the punchline.

Soon enough, we ourselves had joined the crowd, and made our way up bustling Columbus Avenue, past a Chinese street orchestra making strange, beautiful music, to the fabled City Lights Bookstore. As the others went in, I stood outside for four or five minutes, to prolong the moment, to just stand on that sidewalk in front of that doorway. City Lights isn't merely a shrine, of course. It's also a working independent bookstore. The four of us browsed separately for the next hour, occasionally encountering each other, but not really speaking, each engrossed in our own experience. I was determined to buy a book by Kerouac, money be damned, if my debit card would pass muster. Alpha by author, right? But every time I got to the K's, it skipped right over K E R O U A C. I looked to the right of Kerns. I looked to the left of Kerr. No Kerouac. I looked to the *left* of Kerns and the *right* of Kerr, just to be sure. Kerouac was missing. Missing from the shelves of the City Lights Bookstore! There wasn't even a blank space where his books should have been. Perplexed and alarmed, I moved to another section, and another, and then returned. Still missing! I found Joe in the basement, immersed in anarchist literature. He waved me off, deeply engrossed, when I began to express my alarm about the missing Kerouac. I perused every section of the basement, first and second floors, keeping an eye out for Kerouac, but he was gone, man, gone. At the north end of the store, on the street level floor, in an old foyer around the base of a stairway, my eyes fell upon a small hand-lettered sign: "Beat writers on the third floor." I took the stairs, two steps at a time. There was Kerouac, Ginsberg, Ferlinghetti, Snyder, Burroughs—and Laura, deep in browse mode, along with a dozen or so other pilgrims. I bought Kerouac's "Dharma Bums," and Ginsberg's "Howl". The cash register held me in suspense for several seconds as it considered whether to accept my card, which it did after due diligence.

"Hey, Joe," I said, as we all climbed Nob Hill on the way back to the hotel, "Elliott Bay, Powell's, *and* City Lights! We're now members of the West Coast Literati, eh? Hey, let's rename this expedition, 'Books Without Borders!' Get it? See what I did there? Books without *Borders*?" I burbled on in this happy, inane manner until we got to the hotel.

We congregated in Laura and Annie's room, but after a couple of minutes I slipped out. I was eager to read, and just lounge alone for a while. I pulled the curtains open in my room, settled into a chair by the window, and opened "Howl". After twenty lines, my eyes drifted up from the book and out the window, as I vividly remembered the "angelheaded hipsters," and the "screaming vomiting whispering facts" of my youth. I let my memories carry me back.

Out of the Frying Pan

The Saturday after my twentieth birthday, I shaved carefully, dabbed on a little Brut, hiked through downtown Richmond, past the library, past the courthouse with its World War II tank on the lawn and its Armed Services recruiting station, past the jail, and over the bridge to the west side, to Earlham. Earlham's campus was beautiful in spring. The girls had shed their winter coats, and strolled in clusters, showing off their legs. Shirtless boys ran through them, diving after Frisbees. I began spending more of my free time there. By the end of the month, I'd taken a deep breath, gathered up all my records, filled out the confusing and tedious forms, as best as I could, and made an appointment with an Earlham admissions counselor.

I glanced nervously around his small office after he'd shaken my hand and invited me to sit. There were shelves filled with books in disarray. Framed certificates hung on the walls, along with a couple of personal photos, and an institutional clock. His desktop held stacks of loose papers, a big coffee cup, a clean ash tray, a rack of smoking pipes, and the current Rolling Stone issue, with Marvin Gaye and Hubert Humphrey sharing the cover. His window offered a view of the quad, and filled the room with light.

Once I'd sat down, and looked at his face, his horn-rimmed glasses, and his sandy beard, I realized that he was the man with the sandy beard who'd been sitting on Christine's sofa, when I'd knocked desperately on her door in mid-winter, and been sent on my way. If he recognized me, he never let on. He asked me why I'd selected Earlham, and what my academic interests were. I told him how I loved Earlham, and said something vague about wanting to learn about things. He nodded rapidly as I spoke. Then he perused my documents.

When he got to my high school transcript, he looked at it for a long time. Then he turned it over to look at the back, which was blank. That seemed to disappoint him. He looked up at me, set all my papers aside, and told me, not unkindly, that I had not been academically prepared to succeed at their institution, and my success was his goal. He advised me to enroll at the local community college, get a two-year associates degree in liberal arts, and then come back and re-apply at Earlham, with a specific course of study picked out. At which time they would give my application every consideration.

We rose, he handed me back my documents, we shook hands, and he walked me out to the hallway. Outside, with my papers clamped under my arm, and my head bowed, I trudged past his window, and off the campus. Halfway across the bridge, I stopped, flung my papers over the side, and watched them loosen and take flight.

I trudged past the jail, and past the courthouse. Then, without understanding my actions, or wanting to, I turned around, entered the courthouse, and stepped into the recruiting offices. I asked to speak with the Air Force recruiter.

If I had chosen the Army or Marines, my training would have included crawling through mud and barbed wire while men screamed insults, after which training I'd be shipped to a steamy jungle, where I'd be expected to shoot people on demand. The Navy, also, didn't appeal to me. I imagined months of claustrophobic tedium aboard a ship, and then being targeted, a thousand miles from land, by planes and missiles determined to destroy and sink us. So, I joined the Air Force. I liked their sharp blue uniforms, and they got to fly around in airplanes, which I found very appealing.

The friendly recruiter, resplendent in dress blues, rose crisply and offered his hand. We introduced ourselves, and he invited me to sit.

"How old are you, Richard? May I call you Richard?"

"Yeah, sure. I'm twenty."

"Why do you want to join the Air Force, Richard?"

"Seems like I've reached a kind of dead end around here."

"There's a war on, you know."

"I could use the distraction."

He laughed and leaned back in his chair. "Assuming you qualify for acceptance into the United States Air Force, Richard, what field would you like to go in to?"

"Whattaya got?"

I could choose three from among the many job opportunities they had to offer. One would be my preferred choice, and the other two would be back up plans, in case I wasn't qualified, or in the event there were no available slots when the time came. At last, someone was offering me multiple choice career decisions! My first choice was electronics, which I'd been told was the wave of the future. My second choice was medical technician. I don't remember my third choice.

He was very helpful with the paperwork. All I had to do was fill out a couple of questionnaires, and sign a couple of forms, and he would take care of the rest of it. He then confirmed for me that the U.S. government, out of sheer gratitude for my wartime service, would pay for my college education once I returned to civilian life and enrolled at the college of my choice. They might even help me with that paperwork, too, he further assured me, with a smile and a wink.

I didn't get to go into electronics in the Air Force. I failed a color-blindness test, which came as quite a shock to me. I couldn't be trusted to read the color-coding on aircraft wiring harnesses.

I remember arriving at Lackland Air Force Base, in San Antonio, Texas, for basic training. Thousands of recruits had converged there from all over the country. We were herded into a building wearing civilian clothes and various hairstyles. When we emerged, we were all wearing identical uniforms and hairstyles. As each of us came out, we were supposed to get into formation with the men we went in with. There were dozens of formations. I couldn't recognize anyone, so I didn't know which group to fall in with. A sergeant was standing near me, so I approached him and, wearing my best winning smile, asked for assistance. This sent him into a rage. He screamed at me, nose to nose, for two or three intense minutes. He ordered me to never smile at him, or anyone else, ever again. This might be due to the training I later received, but I still remember his dental work. He had gold caps on the molars in his lower right quadrant.

After basic training in San Antonio, Texas, I was sent up the road to Sheppard Air Force Base, in Wichita Falls, for a course in basic medical fundamentals. We learned how to take vital signs, how to give cpr to a dummy, and we role-played in a simulated plane wreck disaster for triage training.

Since we were in the "armed forces", and there was a war going on, we were also given firearms training. One day they bussed us out to a firing range. We spent an hour or so assembling and disassembling over and over again an M-16 rifle. Then they marched us outside and stationed us along a firing line. Each of us had a target about a hundred feet in front of us and twenty rounds of ammunition. They had us lie on our bellies, get comfortable and fire our twenty rounds into our targets when ordered.

After the gunfire stopped, they gathered our weapons and had us fetch our targets. They examined everyone's target and counted the bullet holes. When one of the sergeants counted the score of the man next to me, they found 40 bullet holes in his target. Two other sergeants came over and checked his count. They came up with similar numbers. How could he have hit the target 40 times with 20 rounds? The mystery was solved when they turned around and looked at me. The target I held was still in like-new condition. Not a single bullet hole. This gave the appearance that I might have been aiming at the wrong target.

"Airman, what the hell?" they demanded, gathering around me. "Color-blindness?" I offered. The sergeants didn't have time for this kind of confusion on their reports. After a quick conference, they awarded each of us 20 points and moved on, laughing among themselves. If I remember correctly, I was later given a ribbon for marksmanship, before being shipped to my duty station.

I was assigned to work as a dental assistant in the dental clinic at Langley Air Force Base, headquarters of the Tactical Air Command, in Hampton, Virginia.

Enroute to Langley, I had a few days leave, so I went home to visit my parents. The look of pride on both their faces when they saw me in my crisp, blue uniform, and my shined shoes was unmistakable, though unspoken. I'd also put on ten pounds of muscle from the physical training, and unlimited food supply. I visited with a couple of my old cronies while home, but only a couple. I spent most of my time with my family.

Most of the dentists at Langley were just out of dental school, and just out of officer training, their Captain's bars shiny and new. Uncle Sam had paid for their schooling in exchange for four years of their professional services in the Armed Forces. As a group, they all acted as if they were auditioning as extras in the tv show M.A.S.H., when it came to military bearing, but they were earnestly dedicated to practicing their new skills as dentists.

It was an easy, interesting job, with good hours: 8 to 5, Monday through Friday, and one Saturday per month on call. I had to make coffee one morning each week, and buff the floors one evening each week (these were rotating responsibilities among the low-ranking airmen). I spent my workdays shining a light into peoples' mouths, and handing tools to dentists. There's a whole world in there, among the teeth and gums.

When I wasn't at work, the social scene among the airmen came as a shock to me. I suppose I'd expected us all to be as wholesome as we'd been forced to look, with our haircuts and starched uniforms. I'd figured on the occasional party, the occasional crazy drunken spree, the occasional joint or two. I was wrong. Back home, my peers and I had experimented with drugs out of curiosity, for the most part, and for sensory pleasure, and to try to be cool. I'd grown sick of all of that, and that was why, among other reasons, that I'd enlisted. But I'd leaped out of the frying pan and into the fire, as they say. In the Air Force, getting high was an act of defiance among those of us at the bottom of the pecking order. The peer pressure was relentless. You were either "cool", meaning that you smoked pot when pot was being smoked, or you were "not cool", meaning that you were shunned. You weren't one of "us", you were one of "them", meaning the thick-wasted career sergeants who told us what to do. It was all very depressing.

There were good times and bad. We spent Saturdays at Buckroe Beach, and some weekends down the coast at Cape Hatteras, home of Kitty Hawk. I loved that whole string of barrier islands. In those days, the cape was a one-hundred mile long broken strand of beaches, sparsely settled by small villages catering to the tourists. I don't want to ever go back. I love my memory of it too much. I really can't imagine that it hasn't since been spoiled by too many people and too much development. I remember body-surfing, I remember how slowly the sun rose over the ocean (it seemed to be an event that lasted hours). I remember the little seafood bars. And girls, of course. And sweet southern soul music chugging out of the jukeboxes.

There were epic poker games ongoing back on base, in the barracks. There were loud, deranged parties in off-base rented houses. A lot of airmen were returning from Viet Nam, and most of them had purchased, for ridiculously small sums, top of the line stereo systems. Sansui, and Yamaha, were big names at the time, and we turned them up loud.

But when the noise died down, when the song ended, and the high wore off, when I'd closed the door to my room, then the dark, merciless introspection returned to fill the quiet. Peoples' faces sometimes looked strange to me, including my own. I remember sometimes catching sight of my own hands, my own arms, and they seemed as if they weren't mine. They seemed somehow further away from me than they should be. I remember fleeting incidents of hearing the words I was speaking, and, although they sounded identical in every way to the words I'd always spoken, they'd been hollowed out, drained of content. How is that possible? How can you utter the word "lamp", for instance, and not conjure up the image of a lamp? I began to withdraw.

I remember carrying a chair from my barracks room up the fire escape to the flat roof on summer nights. The barracks were three stories high. From up there, I could sit and look out over Langley from a comfortably detached distance. I could see the magnolia-lined streets where the officers lived on-base in a military-issue mock-Tudor neighborhood. I could see the flightline, where fighter jets frequently flew in and thundered off in squadrons (temporarily drowning out Pink Floyd's "Dark Side of the Moon", which was always, as I recall, being pumped out from one or more barracks window by somebody's powerful stereo). On the other side of the runway was a restricted area where NASA, and others, did secret things in wind-tunnels. I had my own secret, which grew in me, as I sat up on the roof with the world at bay.

Hiding in the Woods

There wasn't a distinct moment when I decided to go AWOL. Over several months, the internal conversation gradually turned from "whether" I should do it to "when". Eventually, I realized that there is no right time to do a wrong thing. If I waited for the right time, then I'd never do it. Once I realized that, I just waited until a convenient payday, drew my pay, filled up a backpack with necessaries, put on good boots, walked off-base and stuck out my thumb. I headed for the Great Smoky Mountains.

I don't recall the getting there, just the being there. Once in the park, I shunned the road, and followed instead a slender bankside path upstream along the Little Pigeon. I climbed all the way up to where the stream comes unbraided, somewhere in the deep shade of Mt. Leconte. When it grew dusk, I rolled out my sleeping bag among the ferns and rested in the cave-like darkness of the deep woods at night, listening to the sound of water running all around me. I never got sleepy, so I laid there listening until morning. When I came out of my bag, I found that the silent dew had soaked its outside, along with everything else.

Light filtered down through the Fraser Firs, Sugar Maples, Buckeyes, Witch-Hazel, Rhododendrons, and Mountain Laurel, to my hiding place in the ferns, as I nibbled on a chunk of greasy cheddar cheese and a Hershey bar. When it was warm enough, I bathed. I dried on a rock in a small pool of light. I boulder-hopped upstream and down. That afternoon, I ate a bologna and cheese sandwich.

Next morning, after another night awake, I ate the last of my food, although I wasn't hungry. I occasionally heard the distant hum of a car on the road that went up to the pass. The unwelcome sound caused me to stand still in deep shadows and listen until it had gone. I clambered up Alum Cave Creek, and took the Styx Branch, up the steep side of Mt. Leconte. The water grew smaller but wilder. I lay down by a slender waterfall but it was too noisy, so I moved back downstream until it got too dark to walk in the thickets. I lay down in a quiet, mossy spot. I listened through the night to furtive rustlings, and small snappings around me. Once, I heard heavy footfalls and a splash as something crossed the stream below.

I spent much of the next day lying on my belly on smooth boulders, studying the fish. They flashed as they turned in the deep pools. When I felt empty, I drank the cold, sweet water.

The next morning, I woke up in daylight, surprised to find that I'd been asleep. I sat up slowly. After a while, I got on my feet. My legs were unsteady. My head was wet with the morning dew. I walked over to the cold, rushing water, sank to my knees in the mud and moss, and dunked my head. When I came up, gasping, I heard a car door slam, and voices.

I scrambled back to my bag and pack, dragged them behind an oak tree, rolled up the bag, secured it onto the pack, and lifted them onto my back. I stood still, listening. Voices calling, laughing, upstream. I fled downstream, my heart racing.

Once I was on the move, I stayed moving, sometimes along the streamside path, sometimes not, but staying along the pounding river, which seemed to be fleeing along with me. When I got into briar patches, down in the bottoms, I pushed straight through them. Thorns tore at my arms, my hands, my bare chest, and my face, but I didn't slow down. I welcomed the burn, the sting, the small bloody ribbons. "Haaaaaahhhh! Haaaaahhhh!" I cried above my panting breath. It was a kind of ecstasy.

Once I got to the edge of Gatlinburg, still following alongside the stream, I calmed down by necessity, washed my cuts, put on a t-shirt, climbed up onto the roadway, and walked into town. I stepped into the first café I saw, and took a booth, my pack and I sitting side by side, like two flayed companions. The waitress stopped about five feet away. "Drank?" she asked, from her safe distance.

"Coffee." My voice was a dry mumble. It sounded like somebody else.

"Water?" she asked, backing away to get the coffee.

"No, I'm good."

When she set the coffee down delicately in front of me, I ordered two cheeseburgers with everything, French fries, peach pie ala mode, and a glass of milk.

On the Lam

I hitchhiked home. Again, I don't remember getting there, just being there. I remember how no one asked any questions when I showed up at my parents' home unexpectedly. And, when I didn't leave after a few days, and then a few weeks, and then a few months, still, no one asked me any questions. At first, they were too discreet to ask, too decorous. And then, there was no need to ask because the answer was self-evident. I had gone awol, after a year in the Air Force. I got my old apartment back, to my surprise, and began to hang out with some of my old cronies.

I found day-to-day work as a temporary laborer through Manpower. On my application, I replaced a 5 on my social security number with an 8, and changed my middle initial from an L to a J, hoping that it would throw the government hounds off my trail. But I could feel them coming after me. I knew my name was being delivered from inbox to outbox, desk to desk, department to department, in an unhurried path to the unknown person who would, one day, be dispatched to retrieve me. By fall, my feeling of apprehension had begun to wear on me. I was watchful all the time. People told me I seemed jumpy. One evening, I went to a party at Little John's apartment, and saw, for the first time in over a year and a half, my old acquaintance, Cliff. He'd put on weight and gone soft. He'd lost more teeth. He tried to sell me some Quaaludes.

"Hell, I was just kidding," he said, after I'd declined. "Just my way of saying hello. I know that's not your thing, and I don't have any anyway. So, I hear you're awol," He was the only person who'd had the nerve to say those words to me. We were sharing a bong.

"Yep." I choked on the bong hit.

"How come?"

"Too many drugs in the Air Force. I came home to clear my head."

He chuckled. "So, you just gonna hang around here 'til they come get you?"

"No. I'm thinking of splitting, actually." It was true. I hadn't told anyone else.

"Where to?"

I looked around to make sure no one else at the party was listening. "Denver."

"When?"

"Payday." It was time to move. I could feel them getting closer.

"Cool. I'll go with you."

I just looked at him for a second or two. "Dude, I'm going out there to disappear. Two guys can't get rides. Forget it. In fact, forget that I even told you."

"I got a cousin in Boulder who'll put us up."

"I don't think so."

"I got six hundred dollars says you do. How much you got?"

"Two hundred."

"What are we waitin' for, stud?"

"Cliff, why do you even want to go? You weren't even thinking about it until just now."

"Been waitin' for the right opportunity. I need to disappear, too."

"Okay, but what do you need me for?"

"How will I know I've really disappeared, if no one's there to see it?"

He wouldn't take no, and six hundred dollars was pretty persuasive, so, after a while, I agreed to let him travel with me. Then I told him the truth: "I'm not really going to Denver, Cliff. I'm really going to Florida. You still interested?"

He shrugged. "Whatever. I got a cousin in Tampa who'll put us up. Why'd you say Denver?"

"like I said, I need to disappear. I need to cover my tracks. So, here's how I want to do this: we tell everybody we know, between now and payday, that we're going to Denver. Then, we go to Florida instead. No one, and I mean no one, knows where we're going, except for the two of us. Agreed?"

He grinned. "Agreed."

By the time the party was over, we'd announced that we were hitch-hiking to Denver in a few days. "Rocky Mountain high, man!" Cliff shouted, raising his glass.

I told my family I was going to Denver. I told my landlady I was going to Denver. I told my boss at Manpower I was going to Denver. I even asked for the address of the local office in Denver. Then, once I'd cashed my check, Cliff and I met up, made a cardboard sign, "TAMPA, FL.", got a ride to the highway from my friend, Little John, and stuck out our thumbs.

It was already late afternoon by the time we left Richmond, but it didn't matter when we began. We were young, we had no futures, and we'd shrugged off our pasts. Our worldly possessions were on our backs, and in-cluded shelter, fire, food and water. Anything else we needed would come to us, we were sure, from the people we were bound to meet along the way. For protection, we each had a knife hanging from our belts, discreetly positioned around to the back. I had a couple of paperbacks, and Cliff had a deck of cards. What few other possessions I'd cobbled together in my short life, I'd either abandoned in Virginia, or stowed away in a closet at my parents' house. Ten miles a day, or a thousand. It didn't matter to us. We could stop and make camp almost anywhere.

Hitchhiking is a leap of faith, for both parties. Successful hitchhiking required the honing and application of a specific set of skills. You only have about three seconds to make an impression on a passing driver, so everything has to be done right, to lure them to pull over. A sign is always a big help. It tells passers-by something about you. If they know where you're going, they can imagine themselves fitting in to your journey, and you into theirs. You want to look like a happy-go-lucky rover, with stories to tell that might free them for a little while from the constraints of their own routines. It's important to look the driver in the eye as he passes. That helps make you less anonymous. If they're wavering, that eye-contact can seal the deal—as long as you don't appear challenging, or desperate. You also need, if you can, to stick out your thumb for each passer-by, individually. That, along with the eye-contact, is a personal request for assistance, from you to him.

A lot of young people were out there along America's highways with their thumbs out, and a lot of people were willing to stop and give them a ride, in those optimistic days, following the idealistic 60's. With luck and skill, we could sometimes get across the country in about the same amount of time it would have taken to drive our own vehicles.

Then, as now, two or more men hitchhiking together raised the number of hitchhikers arithmetically, but it decreased the possibility of success exponentially. Especially when one of the hitchhikers was unaware of, or indifferent to, the necessary skill-set, and liked to lay down beside the road with his head on his pack, one ankle crossed over the other knee, and his arm rising and falling with as little effort as possible as cars and trucks sped past. A man, that is to say, like Cliff.

Maxwell Greenfield

Our first ride, eastbound on I-70, got us to the intersection of I-70 and I-75, north of Dayton. We intended to take I-75 south all the way to Tampa. We stalled out for a couple of hours at the intersection. Finally, about sundown, our second ride got us through Dayton, and on to the outskirts of Cincinnati. Again, we stalled out. We were in a thickly settled suburb, so camping there was likely to be a bleak night under a bridge. Finally, just as we were about to give up for the night, our third ride stopped, and they got us through Cincinnati, across the Ohio River, and just a few miles into Kentucky, somewhere near the town of Florence. We had just climbed out of the car, gotten our packs onto our backs, and were peering into the surrounding darkness for a place to sleep, when a 1966 Plymouth Valiant whooshed by and then screeched to a stop fifty feet beyond us. As we were running up to it, the driver's door flew open, the driver clambered out, wheeled around in a circle, bent over, and vomited all over his left front tire.

By the time he'd finished, and stood upright again, we had arrived at his side. Glancing at us, he took the last swig from a pint bottle of whiskey, washed it around in his mouth for a couple of seconds, and spit it out onto the same tire. "What a waste," he muttered, wiping his mouth and chin with his tie, and letting the empty bottle fall onto the pavement, with a soft clink. "Thank you, boys," he said, as he pushed past us to open the backdoor to his car. "Keys are in it," he called out over his shoulder, as he climbed into the backseat. "We're goin' to Nashville. Jus' follow the signs. Wake me when we get there."

Grinning at each other, Cliff and I stuffed our packs into the backseat beside him, and climbed into the front seat. I took the wheel, and off we went. The air inside the car was so alcohol-infused it made my eyes water. The man's wallet lay on the dash, swollen as a snakebite.

By the time I'd made highway speed, our host was snoring loudly. His snores were mixed with occasional bouts of laughter. "Nashville. How far's that?" Cliff wondered aloud. I looked over at him. He was staring at the wallet on the dash.

"Don't know. A pretty good ways, I think. Nashville. Cool."

"Cool."

After about 20 minutes, the snoring stopped abruptly, mid-snore. "Son of a bitch!" we heard from the backseat. Then, "Hah! Found it." A fifth of Jack Daniels, about three-quarters empty, was thrust forward into the space between Cliff and me. "Hoo-wee! Howdy, boys! Help yourselves."

Cliff took the bottle, drank deeply, and offered it to me. I waved it off.

"My name's Maxwell Greenfield. What might y'all's be?"

"Johnny," I lied, instinctively. Maybe, I had a feeling of what was coming.

Cliff, picking up my cue, also lied. "Jim," he said.

"Johnny and Jim! Well, I can tell you're a couple of fine fellers. I appreciate you drivin'. I was gettin' kinda sleepy. Where the hell are we anyway?"

"We just passed Walton, and coming up Crittendon," I answered.

"Son of a bitch! I thought I told you boys we're goin' to Nashville!"

"You did," I replied.

"Well, you missed your turn! S'posed to turn at Walton. Take seventy-one."

"Guess I missed it. Sorry. You mean Nashville isn't on seventy-five?"

"Oh, hell no."

"Well, that's out of our way, then. We're going down seventy-five, to Florida."

"Florida? I don't know why anybody'd want to go to Florida, but if you get me to Nashville, you'll still be a bunch closer than you are now. I reckon we can turn at Lexington, cut over to Elizabethtown and down. Son of a bitch. Stick with me, boys. I'm too damn tired to drive."

"What do you think?" I asked Cliff.

"Hell, 'Johnny', let's go to Nashville." He was still staring at the wallet.

"Hoo-wee! Boys, just look at that moon." He pointed at a Gulf station sign up ahead.

"That's a Gulf station sign," I said.

"Well, pull in there, then. I just remembered, I gotta piss like a Kentucky thoroughbred. Which is what I am, boys. What I am, what I am."

I took the exit, pulled up to the building, which was open all night, and parked. Maxwell Greenfield struggled out of the car, ineffectually smoothed his disheveled suit, and slowly navigating to the service station door, with a few missteps along the way. He pushed the door. It didn't budge. After a moment of confusion, he pulled it, and it flung open.

Cliff and I were sitting in his car with the engine running. Greenfield's wallet was so stuffed with bills it wouldn't fold. We looked at each other.

"You thinking what I'm thinking?" Cliff asked.

"I don't know. What are you thinking?"

"Same thing as you. Let's do it."

"It'd be so easy, wouldn't it? Just put it in gear, back out, and head down the road."

"We gotta do it now. Put it in gear."

"What does he know about us?"

"Shit. He's so drunk he won't even remember he picked us up."

"He knows we're going to Florida."

"There must be two thousand dollars in there, if there's a penny. Let's go, man! This is our opportunity! It'd be wrong to turn this down. It's a gift!"

I took a deep breath, put the car in gear, and backed out of the parking spot.

"Hoo-wee!" Cliff yelled as I accelerated across the lot.

I took another deep breath and reconsidered. "Cliff! I can't do it! I'm turning around." Instead of turning out onto the road, I circled around in the lot and pulled back to our parking spot.

"You son of a bitch! No! Are you nuts?" As I pulled to a stop, Cliff continued, calling me names, questioning my manhood, and making idle threats, all of which he stopped abruptly when Greenfield came tottering out of the building in his disheveled suit, all smiles.

I was still breathing heavily, and my heart was pounding, as he struggled back into the car. "What're you waitin' for, boys! Let's go to Nashville. I got a girlfriend waitin' for me there, Erma Dean, she's got a head o' hair like Marie Antoinette, and she moves like Little Sheba. She's got a couple daughters, too. You get me to Nashville, I'll introduce y'all."

Cliff slumped down in his seat and closed his eyes. "Nashville's out of our way, Mister," he mumbled. He took a swig of whiskey.

"Nashville *is* the way, boys! Hand me that bottle, lad." Cliff handed him the bottle. He took a drink. "Say, you boys lookin' for work? 'Cause I think you're just the fellers I've been lookin' for. I make a lot of money, and I mean a lot of money, sellin' storm windows, but I got way more business than I can handle. I need some help. I been lookin' for just the right young men to take under my wing. Teach 'em my secrets. If you're the men I think you are, you'll be in tall cotton in no time. But we gotta get to Nashville. My gal's waitin', and so's the president of the company. I got a meeting with him, right after I finish my business with my gal. Y'all don't have anything against makin' money, do you?"

"Well, no," I replied. "It just wasn't in our plans."

Cliff remained silent.

"Plans change, boys. Opportunity knocks."

"No shit," Cliff mumbled.

"These here storm windows? They sell themselves. We use the same glass as the company that makes the glass for the President's limousine, and that's no shit. And the frames? We use a secret alloy that's light and strong. I can't tell you, not yet, what it's made of, but I will say this: NASA. That's all I can say. I got appointments with homeowners lined up for the next two months, and the phone's still ringin'. I take you boys on, you'll have money just fallin' out of your pockets."

"I'd rather go to the beach," Cliff mumbled.

"So, go to the beach! You'll be your own boss. Once you get a few thousand banked up, give yourself a vacation. Course, I'll have to give you an advance to get you started. You'll need new clothes."

"Huh. How about a drink?" Cliff reached back for the bottle. Greenfield handed it to him.

"Drink to the future, lad!"

Cliff drank, but he didn't say to what. As for me, the future was starting to sound pretty good.

"Lord God, I'm tired," Mr. Greenfield continued. "Too tired to drive tonight."

"I'm getting pretty tired myself," I said.

"Keep drivin', son. You can rest when we get there. I keep a suite at the Capitol Hotel. Good mattresses, and a stocked liquor cabinet. Just help yourselves. They make a good breakfast in the restaurant. Just put it on Maxwell Greenfield's tab. They love me there. Cause I know how to tip." He laughed then, as if he'd made a private joke.

Cliff and I looked at each other thoughtfully.

"Did I tell you boys about Erma Dean's twin daughters yet? They're about your ages. Couple o' firecrackers. They'll remind you of Wanda Jackson, before she turned country. And, son, that's a good thing. They're cocktail waitresses in the wildest club in Nashville. Imagine that boys: twin cocktail waitresses. I think they'd like you. They're real easy to please. You like cocktail waitresses?"

As a matter of fact, we did.

"I've just got to close my eyes. Promise me boys. Promise me you'll turn at Lexington. Wake me when we get to Nashville. Lord God ... ." He was snoring within thirty seconds. Within a few minutes, Cliff fell asleep against his door. I was tired, too, but their combined snoring kept me awake. I turned at Lexington.

When we arrived at the outskirts of Nashville, it was just after dawn and overcast. I woke Mr. Greenfield up. Yawning and groaning, he directed me to the Capitol Inn. It wasn't what I'd expected. I'd expected a hotel. This was a motel. I just wanted to sleep, so I didn't say anything. Cliff roused, we got our packs out of the backseat, and Greenfield settled into the driver's seat.

"You fellers get checked in, get some rest. I'll be by this afternoon, and we'll talk about your futures. Just tell 'em you want the Maxwell Greenfield suite, that's number 213, and that I'll be by later. Thanks, boys! Don't drink all my liquor!" He pulled away, laughing.

Nashville

"We need the key to the Maxwell Greenfield suite, number 213, please." There were two women behind the counter. One had risen when we came in.

"Huh?"

I repeated myself. The other woman joined the first. "Huh?" she said.

The Capitol Inn didn't have any suites. None of their rooms had a number that began with a two, since they only had one floor. They'd never heard of a Maxwell Greenfield. They did have vacancies, which we were welcome to rent, but they'd have to charge us for two nights, since we were there so early before normal check-in.

"Huh?" Cliff and I replied in unison. They repeated themselves. We didn't have anywhere else to go. We were dog-tired. We told them we'd take a room.

"How many beds?"

"What the hell's that supposed to mean?" I asked.

"Two?"

"Yeah. Two."

When we paid, I found out that the six hundred dollars Cliff had told me he'd have, was closer to sixty dollars.

"The son of a bitch scammed us!" Cliff said, lying back on his bed, looking at the ceiling and shaking his head.

"No shit. And you both scammed me. Six hundred dollars, huh?" We snapped at each other for a few minutes until we both passed out.

I woke up hungry about five o' clock that afternoon. Cliff didn't stir. At the restaurant next door, I had a big breakfast. I've always enjoyed having breakfast for supper. Not sure why. After I ate, I stepped outside, chewing on a toothpick, and looked around. We were at the city's edge. The motel, restaurant, and other businesses lined a city street. There was a bus stop nearby. But the street was an isolated strand of urbanity. Behind the motel, and around to its north, were undeveloped rolling hills, with patchy wood-lots, and tallgrass pastures. The grass was all winter browns and grays. Small patches of snow lay in shadows. The air temperature felt like it was in the upper 30's, which was pleasantly mild for a northern boy like me. Especially for November.

A couple hundred yards behind the motel, at the end of a long, rutted lane, stood a big, old, unpainted house, surrounded by three or four smaller outbuildings, leaning at different angles. It was picturesque, like a long-abandoned plantation. I walked down the lane. The house had two stories, and a wraparound porch. The yard was as wild as the surrounding prairie, with tall grasses and weeds. There was a pump in the yard. The house and outbuildings made a little cloistered community. A small, feral apple orchard stood inside a falling-down wire fence with a gate that would never close again. There were shade trees, naked for winter, and a couple of red cedars. The place had clearly been abandoned for years, if not decades. I guessed there were about fifteen rooms. The front door was ajar. I stepped inside and sniffed at the silence. Past the foyer where I stood, I saw a big room with a fireplace. Bits and pieces of plaster littered the floor.

I went back to the motel. Cliff wasn't in the room. I found him at the restaurant, and joined him in his booth. We talked about our next move. Florida had really just been a random choice. Cliff had said he had a cousin in Tampa, but I hadn't believed him, and he hadn't mentioned it again.

Since we were there, maybe we should see what Nashville had to offer.

"Got any cousins in Nashville?" I asked, with a sarcastic grin.

"They're all in jail," he replied, returning the grin.

We obviously couldn't continue to live in a motel. I told Cliff about the house, the "abandoned plantation." Next morning, we checked out of the Capitol Inn, carried our packs down the lane and took up residence in the old plantation. Or, to be specific, one room of the old plantation. It was a big, airy room with a working fireplace. We tore boards off the walls for firewood, and rolled out our packs near the fire. The following morning, I took a city bus downtown and signed up for work at the manpower office.

I got a steady job assignment at a paper warehouse. I was able to get there by city buses. Cliff also signed up at manpower, the following day, and got a series of temporary assignments in different locations. He couldn't always get to the job sites, so his schedule was random. Some days, he just stayed at the plantation. When we were there, we kept a fire going from scrap lumber, and cooked humble meals in Campbell's soup cans.

When there was enough light, I perused Brautigan's poems from "The Pill vs The Springhill Mining Disaster", chuckling to myself, while Cliff played solitaire, or stared into the fire. Also, I indulged in more of Castaneda's thrilling reports from the other worlds that surround us. I believed him at the time.

We tacked up the ace of spades on the wall near the fireplace and practiced knife throwing. I got very good at sticking my knife deep into the wall from twenty feet. Sometimes I got close the ace. Cliff found an old Playboy on a shelf, and pinned up the centerfold. We practiced trying to stick the knife into the wall all around her without touching her sacred flesh. I only recall one conversation from those days, and it was our last one.

While we were playing blackjack on the floor by the fire, I asked Cliff, "Hey, Cliff, you know that time you went to jail a couple of years ago? Before I joined the service? I never heard the story. What happened there?"

"I never went to jail." He studied his cards as he spoke.

"Of course you did. Everybody said you did."

"Well, I didn't."

"Where'd you disappear to, then?"

He thought about it for a while before he answered. "I was in the hospital."

"For that long? Come on, man."

"Yeah."

"What for?"

He thought about it for another while. "For something I shouldn't have done."

I let it drop. He became withdrawn for the rest of the evening. I withdrew, too. It seemed that I'd violated a boundary. The following evening, as he sat wrapped in his sleeping bag, staring sullenly into the fire, I asked, "You okay, man?"

After some time, he answered with a question of his own: "So, tell me, Higgs. How's this all adding up for you?"

Actually, I'd thought things were going pretty well. I was having an adventure. "Alright, I guess."

He nodded, and continued staring into the fire. We spoke no more.

The next morning, after I'd washed my face and hair in cold water at the pump in the yard, before heading out to work, he told me he was staying there that day. "See ya later," I said, as I headed out. When I got back that afternoon, he had disappeared. I never saw him again.

After Cliff disappeared, I had about a week or so of solitude at the plantation, in the evenings after work. I didn't miss the company. We'd been fellow-travelers for a while, but I'd never really thought of us as friends, to be honest. Then, one evening after work, I found that all my worldly goods were gone. My pack, my tent, my food, my books, my clothes. All gone. As I stood on the porch absorbing this turn of events, I saw a white Cadillac come bouncing down the lane. I stood my ground.

A large man got out of the car. He wore a cowboy hat and boots, and a bolo tie. He walked up onto the porch where I stood, looking me in the eye the whole time.

"Hello," I nodded.

He nodded back. "Hello, friend. This is my property."

"Yes, sir. I figured."

"People been seeing smoke from my chimney. First time in a long time."

"Yes, sir."

"You can't stay here."

"Yes, sir. Do you have my stuff?"

"I do. I'll give it back, but you have to clear out. Understood?"

"Yes, sir."

He gave me a ride in his Cadillac out to the end of the lane. I used the bench at the bus stop as a work surface to stuff my clothes and small items into the pack, and to strap my tent and sleeping bag onto the outside. I tied my army-surplus poncho over the pack as a raincover. Then, I sat on the bench beside the pack, and tried to figure out what to do next. When the bus came, I got on it. I had no specific plan where to get off. I'd wanted to disappear, and I had. Even from myself, it seemed.

By the time I'd gotten off the bus at the main terminal downtown, a light, cold rain had begun to fall from the failing sky. It was the evening before payday, so I had just a few dollars in my pocket, not enough for a room. I made my way to the Deadrick Street bridge, where the Cumberland River bends around the east end of downtown Nashville.

I heard music and smelled smoke as I scrambled down the bank and ducked under the bridge. There were nearly a dozen men gathered there. We did not exchange greetings. Several men were sitting around a stinking, smoky fire. One of them had a guitar. When I arrived he was singing and playing 'Chug-A-Lug'. Some of the others sang along, laughing and wheezing, on the chorus.

I shrugged out of my pack and leaned it against one of the bridge piers. Then I took off my coat, made a show of sliding my knife around from my hip to my side, and dug a wool sweater out of my pack. After I'd put on the sweater and my coat, I sat down, huddled against my pack, and looked things over.

Two men off by themselves sat on a tarp together, silently sharing what I took to be their last cigarette. One man with his back to the rest stood at the edge of the rain looking out at the river, smoking a cigarette, like a man standing on his porch. Others sat huddled alone in the darker recesses, their tarps, sleeping bags, rags and blankets drawn around them. Others like them had lain down and seemed to be sleeping. Some were old, some were young, all were thin. Once I'd sized them up, none of them looked like a threat.

We were not a community. We'd been tossed together by happenstance. I imagine that we each felt we didn't belong there among the others.

180

Despite the singing and laughter around the fire, an undercurrent of mutual wariness remained.

When the singer began the Grandpa Jones song, 'Good Ol' Mountain Dew', his audience hollered their approval. After it was over, someone asked him to play 'White Lightning', which he obliged. I sidled up to the fire. No one moved to make a hole for me, so I sat a little behind the circle. As a result, I got more smoke than heat, but still, it felt better to be nearer the fire and music. After he finished 'White Lightning', the singer sang 'Hey, Good Lookin'. Someone pulled out a harmonica and tried to play along, without much success. I joined the others in the chorus, but only at a mumble that no one else could have heard.

Young men with guitars have always made their way to Nashville, ready to play for anyone who'll listen. Some end up at the Ryman, some end up under the Deadrick Street bridge, and some end up under the bridge on their way to the Ryman. Our singer was about my age. He wore a dented cowboy hat, pushed way back on his head, which signified friendliness. He had a black eye. He wore gloves with the fingers cut off. Like the rest of us, he needed a good cleaning up, some dental work, and a few hot meals. He brought the song to a close.

"Play 'Lost Highway'," I called out. The expression that came over his face was like that of someone who'd been overtaken by his pursuer after a long chase. He looked at me over the fire, speechless for a moment, and then said, finally, "I don't know that one."

He looked away from me, and never looked back, as he sang 'Jackson'. I retreated to my bridge pier, dug out my sleeping bag and burrowed into it, fully dressed. If I slept, I slept lightly, and if I dreamed, I dreamed I was where I was.

The morning was clear and cold. There was a thin layer of snow on the ground. Packed and loaded, I walked through downtown to the Manpower office, and drew my pay. I told the woman there that I was moving on. I had a big breakfast while waiting for the bank to open. When it did I cashed my check, found a Laundromat, washed all my clothes, and then went shopping at a western wear store across the street from Ernest Tubb's record store. I bought two new shirts and a new pair of jeans, which I stuffed into my pack. After lunch, I checked into a motel at the edge of the downtown district, near the expressway. I napped and read in my room through the afternoon. As evening came, I showered, shaved, put on my new clothes, and went out to dinner. After dinner, I went to Tootsie's and had a few drinks, after which I staggered back to the motel and crashed for the night.

It was early December. It would have made sense for me to continue south to Florida when I left Nashville the next morning, but once I got onto the expressway, I pointed my thumb north. I wanted to go home for Christmas.

Captured!

I'd been home for just a few days, staying at my parents', when I knocked on my old landlady's door to inquire if my old apartment was available. I'd driven by, and it looked unoccupied.

She opened the door and scowled at me. I remember her pointy glasses and sloppy lipstick. I asked her about the apartment. "Young man, aren't you supposed to be in the Air Force?" she replied.

How did she know that? I'd never told her I'd joined the Air Force. "You didn't see me, okay?" I stammered. I turned away from her door and hurried to my car. They'd been there looking for me.

My mother was working as a motel maid at a gas station/café/motel out by the highway at the edge of town. I was to give her a ride home from work that afternoon, and, having nowhere else to go, I drove there to have a coffee, and to think things over while I waited for her.

Late afternoon was a slow time at the café. There were only four or five customers. I sat at the counter, and ordered a coffee. I sat quietly sipping and trying to decide what to do next. A man came in and took a stool at the counter. We were the only two customers at the counter. There was one stool between us. I knew who he was without even looking at him. He ordered a coffee and waited quietly until it was delivered. After he'd taken a sip, he said to me, quietly, "Richard, are you ready to go?"

I turned to him. He looked as I'd expected he would. Neat. Trim. Conservative. Holding my gaze. Not unfriendly. "Agent Robbins, FBI. You're Richard Higgs."

"I need to give my mom a ride home, and pack my clothes. Would that be okay?"

"Sure. I'll come by in two hours. Will you be there?"

I nodded. "It's in Webster."

"I know." He rose, paid, and left. I felt relieved as much as anything. I no longer had to look over my shoulder, and all my decisions for the foreseeable future were about to be made for me.

When he knocked on my mom's door, she hugged me and went to her bedroom. I was packed and waiting. He got through the arrest formalities as quickly and discreetly as the law allowed. He let me see his handcuffs but didn't use them. On the ride into Richmond, we spoke calmly. I asked him why he'd joined the FBI. He told me he wanted to do good. He said it so simply I believed him.

"It was my landlady, wasn't it, who turned me in," I ventured. It had to be. Within thirty minutes of her seeing me, he'd found me at the café.

He didn't answer. "I thought you'd gone to Denver," he said instead.

I smiled inwardly, as if I'd won something because my ruse had worked. I imagined agents of the Denver office of the FBI scouring the streets of Denver for me while I sunbathed on the beach in Florida.

I spent the next three days in the Wayne County Jail, after which, Fort Benjamin Harrison, in Indianapolis, sent out an MP van with a driver, and two armed guards, who took custody of me and another man. We were handcuffed, and chained to a bench in the van, beside two others. We continued on a route through four or five other jails in surrounding counties, picking up other awolees, and ended back at the fort with a full van.

I spent the next three days in a tiny iron cage at the fort. The cage was just big enough to hold a bunk. There was a narrow space between the bunk and the front of the cage, with barely enough room to stand. Soldiers my own age let me out to eat, under supervision, in a mess hall with other prisoners, and, at prescribed intervals, to go to the bathroom, where I could

184

relieve myself, and, once a day, shower and shave. I was sitting on my bunk on the second day, working hard on suppressing a growing panic, when I saw something that made me smile for the first time in quite a while.

My older brother, Danny, had joined the Army three or four years before I'd joined the Air Force. He'd gone through basic training, and then had been assigned to work in a mess hall at his duty station, which was, I think, at Fort Campbell, Kentucky. As soon as he'd learned to make biscuits, he'd gone awol, and headed home to Richmond. There, in my cage at Fort Benjamin Harrison, I saw his name scratched into the paint of the metal panel on the endwall of the cage, along with other names and profane messages. He'd been in the same cage as me. I wrote my name under his, using a ballpoint pen. Seeing his name distracted me for a short time, but feelings of panic brought on by my tight confinement returned.

Prison

People who deal with suicides recognize three distinctions: suicides, suicide attempts, and suicide gestures. A suicide is obviously a successful ending of one's own life. A suicide attempt is a genuine, but unsuccessful, attempt to end one's own life. A suicide *gesture* is not a genuine attempt to end one's life. It is meant only to give the *appearance* of a suicide attempt. As a false suicide attempt, it is a genuine cry for help.

I created a fourth distinction, there in my cage: a false-suicide-gesture-attempt. My plan was to give the *appearance* of a suicide *gesture*. That is to say, the appearance of crying out for help. But I wouldn't *really* be crying out for help. My real and only motive was escape. I wanted out of the cage.

The guards gave every prisoner a shaving kit, which included what is now an old-fashioned razor, with changeable, double-edged blades. It's hard to believe they did that, but they did. After shaving on the third day, I formed a plan for escape. I removed the razor blade, and carried it back to the cage in my pocket. My plan was to cut my wrist with the razor blade, just enough to draw blood, but not enough to actually endanger myself, and then raise a big fuss. I supposed I'd have to scream or something. I pictured them dragging me out of the cage, conveying me to the fort hospital, bandaging me up, maybe even stitching me up, and then assigning me to the mental ward. In the mental ward, I imagined, security would be lax, and I would escape, never to be caged again.

In the cage, sitting on my bunk, I slipped the razor blade out of my pocket, rolled up my sleeve, picked out a spot on my arm, near my wrist, and pressed. What I learned in the next five minutes, was that, no matter how bad things got for me, I'd never be capable of suicide. I pressed the blade against my flesh with every ounce of strength I had, and never broke the surface, because I was also resisting the push with every ounce of strength. The edge of the razor touched my skin as I fought myself to a draw. When

Then There Is No Mountain

I dropped the blade, and lay back on my bunk, my arm was exhausted, I was covered with sweat, and breathing heavily. I began to shake, so I pulled the army blanket around me and laid there until I'd recovered. I might have considered myself the ultimate failure: I couldn't even succeed at giving the *appearance* of giving the appearance of wanting to hurt myself. In the end, however, I found the whole episode strangely reassuring.

Two guards came, opened the cage, and escorted me out to the lobby. "We can't hold you in the cage for more than seventy two hours, airman," one of them informed me. "That'd be cruel and unusual. Well, cruel anyway. Maybe not unusual." They handed my bags over to me, and handed me over to a pair of muscle-bound deputies from the Marion County Sheriff's Department.

I spent the next four weeks in the Marion County Jail, in Indianapolis, waiting in misery for someone from the Air Force to come get me. I learned something in there that I've never forgotten. Before I went to jail, I'd thought that criminals were a "type", different from us non-criminals. The criminal-type was supposed to be mean, intimidating, dumb, uncouth, and dangerous. The ratio of criminal-types to regular guys, among my fellow-criminals, was about the same as on the outside. Most of the men behind bars are just guys like the rest of us who got on the wrong side of some law or other. There are a hell of a lot of laws, and it would be hard not to break one or two from time to time. Some guys get caught. I don't mean to say whether they should or shouldn't be there, or to minimize whatever crime they may have committed. I just mean that there's no such thing as a criminal-type.

Time stood still for four weeks. My memories are impressionistic: awful food on a tray pushed through a slot. A cellmate talking about his wife and kids. A surprising background of laughter, echoing day and night, from the forty cells in our bay. What was so funny? I never found out.

At last, they took me from my cell, rejoined me with my possessions, and pushed me into the lobby. There stood Sergeant Lyle, from the dental clinic at Langley, standing tall in crisp khakis. He signed for me, pulled a set of handcuffs from off his beltloop, and held them up between us. "Am I gonna need these, Higgs?"

"No way, Sergeant Lyle. I'm just glad to see you. Please, take me back."

We drove to the airport and, boarding a commercial flight, made our way back to Langley, where he turned me over to the base Military Police.

They weren't sure what to do with me. I was sitting in a chair, as instructed, in the base MP station. MPs wandered in and out. Some stood around sipping coffee. Others filled out report forms. Everyone took notice of me. I was an object of curiosity.

"He did what? Went AWOL? Why?" This question kept getting repeated among them.

The desk sergeant called out to me: "Airman! Did you really go AWOL?"

I nodded.

"What the hell?" He replied.

I shrugged.

It's virtually unheard-of for anyone to go AWOL from the Air Force. Langley Air Force Base didn't have a brig. They'd apparently never needed one, until me.

"Says here you worked over at the dental clinic."

I nodded again.

"You went AWOL from that? What the hell?"

I shrugged again. He shook his head in disbelief. "Well, he's in my way," he said to the MPs who'd brought me there. "Put him in the drunk tank, I guess, until we figure somethin' out." I spent the night in the drunk tank–a small room with a cot, and a window with unbreakable wire-glass.

By next morning, they'd made arrangements for me to be transferred to the U.S. Navy brig across Hampton Roads in the Norfolk Naval Base. Before they took me over, Sergeant Lyle came by with a duffel bag stuffed with my uniforms. Once I was back in uniform, the put me in a van and delivered me to the Navy brig, where I waited among the sailors for my court-martial date. I stood out like a sore thumb in my wrinkled Air Force uniform.

At my court-martial, back at Langley a couple of weeks later, I met my military lawyer. When we shook hands, he asked me if they'd been treating me okay. I had no complaints. We sat at a table before the judge. The lawyer opened his briefcase and arranged his papers on the table. It was a perfunctory affair. I pled guilty. Like everyone else, the judge, the prosecutor (if that's his title), and my lawyer all wanted to know why I'd done it.

I shrugged.

They all just waited.

When I spoke, my voice sounded like someone else's. "I got really depressed. I joined the Air Force to get away from home. I went back home to get away from the Air Force. I hadn't been able to figure out where to go. I felt desperate. I'm better now, though."

The judge sentenced me to six months in the brig. My time in the Wayne County Jail, the Fort Benjamin Harrison holding cell, the Marion County Jail, and the U.S. Navy brig, all added up to six weeks of time served. So, I spent the next four-and-a-half months in the brig.

During prisoner orientation, we new prisoners were informed that we were there "as punishment, not for punishment." Evidently, they didn't intend to beat us. We'd be able to take classes in this-or-that if we wanted. We'd have access to medical and mental care, as needed. There would be duty assignments, including working in the laundry facility, grounds maintenance, and other menial tasks. We would be forbidden from wearing pressed or starched uniforms. Our wrinkly uniforms were meant to identify us as prisoners.

I have just a few memories of my time in the brig. I remember endless games of spades. I remember working in the laundry, pressing others' uniforms. I remember softball games in the yard. I was a reliable hitter, and I almost always made it to first base. One softball game in particular stands out. As we were playing, a Lockheed C5A Galaxy came in for a landing at the base, and lowered itself right over our ball diamond as it approached the base runway. It brought the game to a standstill as its enormous shadow passed over us, and its roar drowned out our voices. Its size gave the illusion that it was traveling impossibly slow. How could it hang there in the sky? We looked at each other in wonder.

I remember that there were supposedly two infamous prisoners among us: Two sailors who'd attempted to sell nuclear submarine design secrets to Soviet agents, and had been caught. They were in such *big* trouble, the rest of us, with our petty crimes, spoke of them in whispers—or so my memory tells me. They were being held in a different wing, so none of us ever actually saw them.

I also remember that there was a small library. I discovered a book by Dr. Laurence J. Peter, called "The Peter Prescription", wherein I read about the Peter Principle. The Peter Principle is Dr. Peter's explanation of how people in any hierarchical organization inevitably rise through the ranks, to their level of incompetency, and stop there. As a result, all hierarchical organizations are always being run, at all levels, by incompetents. Since military organizations are the most hierarchical organizations of all, he held them up as the purest exemplars. Considering my situation, It's not surprising that I found it a deeply satisfying read. I don't remember the "prescription"—probably something about how society should evolve to less hierarchical organizations. It was a Sixties thing. I hoped I hadn't yet risen to my own level of incompetency.

I also remember being asked, again and again, "You went AWOL from the Air Force? Why?"

I don't remember any particular desire to escape. Everyone around me was clean and sober. Nobody expected much of anything from us. It was four-and-a-half months of downtime.

Datura stramonium

When I was released back to duty among my old comrades at Langley, I was tan, fit, and rested. The rounds of off-duty partying had continued in my absence, of course, and within a week, I'd unhappily succumbed to the relentless peer pressure to fill my body and mind with pot, hash, and wine. The need to be accepted is a powerful thing.

Among my possessions, when they were returned to me from storage, I found an unfinished paperback of Castaneda's "Tales of Power". I picked up the story where I'd left off, before going AWOL, and was drawn like a moth to images of lean, dark, white-haired Yaqui mystics gathered around fires in the exotic desert night, ingesting strange plants, and then flying through other worlds, other worlds that exist right here around us, and engaging powerful animistic enemies and allies in epic quests, and then returning with the morning, exhausted, their peasant shirts stained with vomitus, and sleeping for 24 hours, after exchanging knowing glances with the crows watching the sunrise from nearby branches. Castaneda swore it was all true, he'd been there, he'd participated. Among other things, they smoked datura, those mystics. I looked it up.

Datura stramonium is also known as Jimsonweed, or, more formally, Jamestown weed. It acquired this popular name because, in the 1670's, several British soldiers, stationed at Jamestown, Virginia, had ingested it, and, for the next eleven days, appeared to have all gone insane. It's also called loco weed. Jamestown was, coincidentally, only a few miles from where I was when I read about this. I studied a botanical drawing of Jimsonweed, and realized that I'd seen it all my life. It was a common weed that sprung up in areas where the soil had been disturbed by construction, erosion, or cultivation.

I found a plant, right there on the base, not far from the clinic. It had white, trumpet-shaped flowers that smelled awful. I gathered leaves and seeds. That weekend, at a big party off-base, in a house that some airmen had rented, I announced that I was going to brew up some Jimsonweed tea and give it a try. I wanted to see God, I said, half-jokingly. I damn near did, before it was over.

I put a pot on the stove, tossed in some dried leaves and crushed seeds, and brought it to a boil. When it had cooled, I poured myself a glass. It had the color of watered-down milk. It was the bitterest, foulest substance I'd ever tasted. I forced it down, and waited, as the party raged on around me. After thirty minutes, nothing had happened. I poured another glass, and forced it down.

I began to see strange figures flitting in and out of my peripheral vision. At first, whenever I turned to see them better, they disappeared, but soon, they were all around me, joining, or supplanting, my fellow airmen. They were, I quickly realized, demons. Those monstrous visions were nothing like the swirling, colorful hallucinations from LSD, which I'd taken a couple of times before. The reason for taking LSD, at least for me, was to marvel at the crazy *un*reality of the experience.

Their gnarled faces, glittering eyes, fangs, and claws were horrifying, and as real-looking as anyone else around me. More real, even. The crystal clarity of every detail of their faces and figures was terrifyingly convincing. They were individualized—each one a different version of horror.

The last thing I remember is sitting in a chair on the front porch, rocking back and forth, as the demons multiplied, and crowded around me. I retreated to an ever-diminishing, hidden niche in my consciousness, where I retained a sense of self and place, and from there I told myself to hold on, to ride it out, it wasn't real, but it was like being strapped to a chair in a rising, boiling flood. The horror rose around me, the demons moved in, and my hiding place became smaller and smaller.

When I opened my eyes, I saw ceiling tiles. Then I saw faces looking down at me. I was groggy, and fell back asleep. When I woke up again, a doctor spoke down to me, and explained where I was. I was in a room at the base hospital at Langley. As I recovered, my doctor, and the couple of visitors who came to see me, told me the story.

I'd flung myself out into the street in front of the house and begun writhing and screaming on the pavement. My fellow-partiers (none of whom had joined me for tea) were afraid that someone might call the cops and bust the party. They tried to drag me back inside the house. I seemed to have developed super-human strength, so they couldn't subdue me. I fled to a neighbor's house. I banged on the door. When the woman who lived there opened the door, I collapsed onto her living room floor, bleeding, howling, crawling in circles, fighting for my life. She called the cops.

It had taken six policemen to subdue me, I was told. I'd been hand-cuffed and rushed by ambulance to the base hospital. When the doctors took my vital signs, they were shocked to find that my temperature was 108.5 degrees. They'd had to take it under my arm. If they'd put a thermometer in my mouth, I'd have chewed it to pieces. They filled a tub with ice, lowered me into it, and sedated me. Someone who'd been at the party told the doctors what I'd taken. They consulted their books, pumped my stomach, concocted and administered an antidote, and waited. They assumed that, in the unlikely event I survived, it would be with permanent brain damage. My temperature dropped, the poison purged, they kept me unconscious for three days before allowing me to surface again.

I was bruised and scarred all over. My wrists were deeply scarred all around, from where I'd struggled against the handcuffs. My thumbs were numb. Sunlight hurt my eyes. I couldn't think straight.

The doctor's seemed to find it hard to believe that they'd saved me. They brought other doctors in to see for themselves. They spoke of alkaloids and atrophine. They scolded me. The day before my release, a doctor I hadn't seen before came to see me. He wanted to know about Jimsonweed. He wondered if I could show him a Jimsonweed plant.

"It's not hard to find. It's just a common weed. You've seen it."

"Show me?"

"Why?"

"Because it's powerful. It might also be a powerful medicine."

I snorted.

"I'm serious. What if all this collapses one day?" He gestured around the room, but he meant *all this*, as in medical science, drug companies, chemical factories. As in civilization as we knew it. "You never know. What would we do for medicine then? I'm interested in organic sources for the medicines we produce synthetically. Will you show me?"

After I was released, we took a walk. I was still a little slow and unsteady. When we got to the dirt mound where I'd found my plant, I pointed it out.

"So, that's it, huh." He approached it. He studied it, turning the leaves over, sniffing the flowers, handling the seed pods. I stayed a safe distance back from it.

I remained spaced out for the next couple of weeks. My peers, as mean and relentless as ever, even knowing what I'd been through, continued to try to force joints on me, which I angrily refused. I just wanted to think straight.

Somehow, I managed to escape my foolish experiment with no brain damage. I had developed a heart murmur, they told me–a "walking" heart murmur, they called it. It must have walked away, because no other doctor has ever detected it in the many years since. My thumbs remained numb for the next two years.

Not long after I'd recovered, I was dispatched to an anonymous office, in a different part of the base, to talk things over with a Captain there. He looked up from my file. "We have a new program. An early-release program.

We think you might qualify." It was the summer of 1974. The Vietnam War had ended. They were downsizing.

"What's the catch?"

"No catch. You'll get an honorable discharge and full veteran's rights. I'm told you're pretty messed up, but not a bad kid. You want out?"

"Where do I sign?"

"Right here."

Discharged

Within a week I was out of the Air Force, and on my way home. Except that I didn't go home. I made my way, instead to Bloomington. It was late August, and I knew that Maggie would be there, to start another year of school, and I needed to see her.

I left Langley about sun-up. Standing outside the maingate, dressed in my summer khaki uniform, beside my duffel bag, I hoisted my numb thumb into the air. My first ride took me to Richmond, Virginia. By late afternoon, I'd gotten past Huntington, West Virginia. Thanks to my uniform, I was making good time. I slept rough in the woods on a narrow shelf of stone up the steep side of a mountain. I had no fire, and didn't need one.

Next day, between Lexington and Louisville, I got a ride from a teen-age couple.

"Welcome home, sir," the boy said to me in his rearview mirror, once I'd gotten settled into their backseat. The girl turned around to look at me. "We're just glad you made it home in one piece," she added.

I didn't know what else to say, so I just said, "Thanks."

"No, thank *you*," the boy replied. "What was it like, over there?"

"Over where?"

"Nam. We supported y'all a hundred percent. What was it like?"

The Vietnam war had been over for a year-and-a-half, but, still, they thought they had a returning hero. How could I disillusion them?

"The horror."

They looked at each other. The girl looked at me. "Was you wounded?"

"They say my thumbs will be numb for the rest of my life."

"Oh my God! What'd they do to your thumbs?"

I shook my head and looked grimly out the window.

"Those rat bastards," the boy muttered.

That night, near Bloomington, Indiana, I slept rough again, in Brown County State Park. When I woke up, I slipped into the campgrounds, where I used the facilities to take a shower and change into jeans and a plaid shirt. I cached my duffel in the woods, and hiked into town to find breakfast and Maggie.

I called my mother and asked her to call Maggie's mother and get a contact number for her. About five minutes after I'd hung up, the payphone rang. It was mom, with Maggie's number. I called Maggie.

We met for lunch, at a pizza place on 3rd Street, across from the campus. She was a half-hour late. She'd changed a lot in the two years since I'd seen her. I saw more of her mom in her face, when she and a guy our age breezed through the door. The guy wore John Lennon glasses, and a wispy attempt at a beard. I'd imagined that she'd come alone. I hadn't imagined I'd feel so nervous. The unwelcome sight of him made it worse.

She hugged me chastely. "Wow. Look at that haircut! I almost didn't recognize you! Rich, this is my fiancée, James. James, Rich, from my hometown. We grew up together. So, you're out, now?"

"Yep. Out for good." My heart sank unexpectedly when I heard her describe me as 'from my hometown.' It meant 'from my past.' Or, worse, 'from my childhood.' It meant she'd placed me among her memories, where I belonged.

James and I shook hands. A little too firmly.

"So, what're you reading these days?" I asked Maggie, as we sat down. She flashed her old, familiar smile at my old, familiar question.

"Wolfe."

"Virginia?" She was a college girl, after all. It seemed a reasonable guess.

"God, no. Thomas."

"Really? Me, too!" I couldn't believe it. Good old Maggie!

"You're kidding! Look Homeward, Angel?"

"No. Electric Kool Aid Acid Test."

"Uh, I don't know that one."

"Oh, you have to read it next, Maggie. It explains everything! Prepare yourself for exclamation points!"

"I'm getting very confused."

James cleared up our confusion by informing us that there is a Thomas Wolfe and a Tom Wolfe, and they have virtually nothing in common. The son of a bitch had read them both. When he took a deep breath to continue his lecture on their respective places in American Letters, I lunged for a menu, prepared to tune him out, but Maggie pre-empted him by asking me if I was still reading Castaneda.

I looked up from the menu. "No, I'm through with all that." Something, I suppose, about the way I said it, must have made her drop the subject. She said no more about it.

Then There Is No Mountain

We had our pizza and beer. We asked each other about the folks back home. They told me about their plans for the future, something about going to Africa, but I was only half-listening, and they asked me about my plans, but I really didn't have any. She told me that Christine had gone to Japan, after all, and that her letters seemed happy.

They lived off-campus with two other couples, and they offered to put me up for the night on the sofa, but I declined. There was a brief, cool embrace, and a quick handshake, when we parted. And that was that. I couldn't have said in words, not even to myself, why I'd wanted to see her, what I might have been hoping for. Hell, I still can't.

I browsed a used bookstore, and picked out a copy of a collection of Stephen Crane's works. I'd found out about him somewhere along the way and had become curious. Then, I stopped in an Army surplus store, where I bought a one-man tent, a lantern, and a cheap backpack to carry them in. On the way out of town, I stopped at a grocery store and bought a lighter, and some sandwich makings for later. That night I paid the fee, and camped at a site in the Brown County State Park campground. I lay by the fire until it went out, and then crawled into my tent and read "The Open Boat", all the way to the end.

Lost in the Corn

I lay in the dark, then, and thought about Maggie. Once, on a late-summer afternoon, the year our parents had met, when Maggie and I were eight years old, our family had gone to visit theirs. Maggie and I had already become fast friends. We liked to play hide and seek in the eighty-acre cornfield that began out behind their barn, so we slipped out into the corn. The corn was far taller than us, the green blades converging over our heads, breaking the sky into shards. That day, the sky was gray. The light that filtered through the corn was soft, and green-tinted. Shadows were indistinct. Nothing grew from that soil but sturdy, close-planted cornstalks. The only other visible living beings, besides us, were a few big, yellow and black striped spiders. Corn spiders, she informed me.

We pushed deep into the field, across the rows. The rows were planted along a curve, so that we could only see down them, to our left and right, twenty or thirty feet in either direction, as the rows converged around the curve. Feeling mischievous, I lagged behind, and then fled down one of the rows as she continued to push through them. I got out of sight before I heard her call my name. My plan was to circle wide around her, and then place myself in her path and surprise her as she came upon me.

But I lost my bearings, and she hers. Our fading voices came to each other from shifting directions, sometimes louder, sometimes softer, absorbed by the corn, obscured by our increasingly desperate thrashing.

When we found each other, seemingly hours later, although it was surely only a few minutes, we were both dirty, sweaty, and scratched by the rough corn. Her face was wet with tears. She hit me in the shoulder with her fist and then sat down, hugging her knees, crying angrily.

"Where'd you go?" she demanded.

"I'm sorry, Maggie," I said, pleadingly.

"Where'd you go?" She repeated. She threw a clod of dirt at me. I let it bounce off my chest, and didn't retaliate. I tried to explain. "Not funny," was all she said.

I sat down beside her. She began to calm down. Since we were eight years old, we didn't hug. "Wow, look at that spider," I said. "Creepy."

"Daddy says they can jump six feet."

"Let's get out of here."

That was a problem. We'd found each other, but we were still lost. We tried backtracking, but our tracks had become so roundabout it was impossible. We felt a rising panic. Then, in sheer desperation, it seems, the solution occurred to me. The rows all ended, in one direction, along the road their house was on. The other direction ended along a fence line that led to an open pasture, from which we could see the house. We set out along the row, to follow it to the end.

A few minutes later, we came out on the road, and walked the couple hundred yards to their driveway. We were home safe. We washed up at a hose in the backyard, and joined our siblings in a game of tag. We hadn't been missed.

"Maggie," I called out softly, in the dark of my tent. "Where'd you go?"

Out of the Dark

When I got to my parent's house, late the next day, I settled into a bedroom, and spent a few days looking for the way forward. During those few days, I spent most of my time with my family, getting grounded.

"You can make a fresh start, now, son," my mom said one morning at breakfast.

She was right! I had an opportunity to re-invent myself. I'd been gone long enough to break old bonds. Who did I want to be, now? There were guys I'd known in school, and in the Air Force, at whom I'd marveled, because they never seemed to look inward. (It was hard to believe, looking back then, that I'd once mistaken Cliff for one of those guys.) They seemed generally happy, and confident, and people seemed to like to be around them. I decided that I'd try presenting myself to the world as one of those guys.

At first it was all false bravado, but a surprising thing happened: after a while, I became what I pretended to be. That's not quite true. I became *more like* what I pretended to be. I turned my gaze outward, forcefully at first, and kept it there, and the world began to open up to me. I locked myself out of certain dark corridors of my soul, and threw away the key. Whenever I felt the urge for introspection, I turned away from it, and engaged the world, and the people around me, instead. After a while, it began to feel natural. I still had an inner life, and there were still times of darkness, now and again, but I'd learned to free myself from their grip.

I went to work for Manpower again, and they kept me busy enough, working for bricklayers, house framers, warehousemen, and others. My most interesting assignment, which lasted several weeks, was to help build a massive pipe organ, with over 5,000 pipes, in one of the local churches. I worked with a crew of happy-go-lucky craftsmen, who'd come in from Hagerstown, Maryland. I'm still proud of that job. I rented an airy apartment in a leafy neighborhood, and the fresh breezes of the world billowed my curtains. Pretty women came, and went, sometimes with no hard feelings.

I took night classes on the G.I. Bill, none of which related to each other, except that they were subjects that interested me: Astronomy, 19th Century American Literature, Anthropology, Algebra, Physics. I made friends among my fellow night-class students. These were adults who were motivated enough to spend their evening hours taking classes, working toward something, or learning about the world, after working all day. I loved being among them. Did my classes add up to a coherent field of study? No, but I didn't care.

Cliff had been right, I realized, when he'd told me that a life isn't supposed to add up to anything. It's not an addition problem, after all. Ironic, I thought, when I further realized that Cliff hadn't really believed it, when he'd said those words to me. How could he have believed it, and done what he did?

I'd been moving in different circles since returning home, so it was several weeks before I happened to run into my old friend, Little John, at the grocery store. He told me that, a few months after Cliff had come back to Richmond, from Nashville, he'd gone to his parents' house one day, when they weren't home. He'd sat down in his father's easy-chair, and stuck the barrel of a loaded pistol into his mouth, and pulled the trigger.

"Why would he do that?" Little John wondered aloud. "It just don't add up."

And so it was, for the next two years. I worked odd-jobs, and took odd classes. But, the confinement of a long, cold Indiana winter stirred up a wanderlust in me, and when Spring came at last, I decided I wanted to see the West, which led to my long summer of cherries and trout.

Leaving San Francisco

I had been gazing absently out the window of my room at the Mark Hopkins during this long reverie, all brought on by reading "Howl". Suddenly, I was brought back to the present by an explosion of color in the sky over the dark bay beyond the city, and then another, and another. San Francisco was celebrating the Fourth of July. On the Third of July. I checked my watch to make sure.

I banged on Laura's room door and brought the three of them back across the hall, where we all pressed our noses to the windows and oohed and ahhed for the next half-hour at the fireworks display. Annie was especially thrilled, being young, and never having seen a Fourth of July fireworks celebration before. A shaped charge exploded into a big red heart above the city. She caught it just right with her cell-phone camera, and immediately sent the image to her boyfriend, Wolf, in Germany. As Paul Simon said, "These are days of miracles and wonders."

As Jerry Reed once observed, we had a long way to go, and a short time to get there. But first, breakfast. But before breakfast, coffee. I dressed, took the elevator to the lobby, found the coffee urn, and settled into one of the expensive-looking wingbacks to sip my morning cup. I refused to look at the newspapers arrayed on the coffee table, choosing instead to watch the well-heeled people gather and go, the sweet rot of old money wafting in their wakes. (My own money is forever young, chasing down the street after the ice cream man.)

After my solitary coffee, I met up with the others. We went out for a quick breakfast and then straight back to the hotel, where we packed up our gear. Laura checked us out at the front desk, and then joined the rest of us in the middle of the crowded lobby. We waited for the hotel staffers to bring the Rover around front and load it for us.

Then There Is No Mountain

Once the Rover was loaded, we plowed a wedge through the kempt women and pink-fingered men, they in their Arminis and Diors, their silks, soft leathers, and linens, and we equally well-draped in our Mountain Hard-wear and First Ascent, our nylon, polyester, and Gore-tex.

Laura wanted to visit Golden Gate Park before we left town, so we headed in that direction, with Joe at the wheel. Without too much trouble, and only a few U-turns and backtracks, we found ourselves driving through the famous Haight-Ashbury neighborhood. I was relieved to find that it has remained comfortably seedy all these years, like the home of a bachelor uncle who washes his dishes once a week and feeds his cat on the counter. (Do you remember him, this uncle of yours? He has a Seventies-vintage component stereo system, including a meticulously maintained turntable, and an immaculate collection of shiny black LPs. A framed Jefferson Airplane poster hangs above his dilapidated sofa, and his rooms smell of sandalwood, coffee, oranges and you-know-what....) Haight-Ashbury seems also to have remained defiantly local in its businesses. We didn't see a Starbucks or Mc-Donald's, nor even a 7-Eleven. Graffiti-embellished headshops, funky second-hand boutiques, and music stores abounded. In our quick drive through, we got no sense of the place having fallen into self-parody.

After a stroll to the Conservatory of Flowers in Golden Gate Park, we re-boarded the Rover, and were then eastbound and down, to quote Jerry Reed yet again. We took I-80 over the Bay Bridge, past Berkeley, El Cerrito, and the city of Vallejo, where I was created. I tried to feel something special when I saw the sign for Vallejo, but neither the sign nor the view gave me anything to work with.

Once past Sacramento, we began to climb out of the Central Valley and up the great wedge of the Sierra Nevada Range. Somewhere near Donner Summit we crossed the Pacific Crest Divide. Donner Summit reminded Joe of a funny story: "Once, my brother, Red, went out on a dinner date with his girlfriend at the time, to this really popular restaurant. The hostess told them it would be about a 25-minute wait, and then she asked for the name of their party. Already hungry, and dreading the long wait, Red replied with a straight face, 'Donner.' They sat down on the crowded bench to wait in misery with the others. About a half-hour later the hostess calls out, 'Donner party! Your table is ready!' That got everyone laughing on the bench."

We crossed into Nevada, and at Fernley we left I-80 and cut over to Fallon, where we got onto U.S. 95 and rolled south toward Las Vegas, our Rover a little black dot rolling down the map. At Hawthorne, we passed the unlikely sight, in that arid desert, of Walker Lake. The route jogs east at Hawthorne, through several miles of earthen bunkers storing the reserve munitions of the Hawthorne Army Depot. About halfway to Tonopah, we occupied ourselves by trying to pick out Boundary Peak, Nevada's highest mountain. We did see a snowcapped peak off to our southwest, and this was July in southern Nevada, so we called that it.

Death Valley

As we passed through Beatty, I was reminded of when Louise and I had surfaced there two summers earlier after driving through Death Valley. It was in July. We'd been up at Yosemite, and we'd decided to cut through Death Valley as we made our way east. There's an overlook on Highway 190 with a view over a section of the deep valley. At the overlook, you are at about 5,000 feet elevation, making the valley floor almost a mile below you. It was early evening. We got out of our pickup to stretch and have a look. The temperature felt like it was in the 60s. The sky was overcast, and it was actually raining, though very lightly. This was not the Death Valley we'd expected. We dropped down into the valley, followed the Nadeau Trail across the floor, then ascended a range, crossed over a pass, and descended again down to Stovepipe Wells, elevation 10 feet.

The sun had set by the time we got there. We parked at the ranger station to check in, as the signs had requested. When I opened the truck door it was like opening the door to a blast furnace. This was so shockingly unexpected that I was dizzy with disbelief as I knocked on the ranger station door. No one was there. A thermometer beside the door registered 108 degrees. When I got back in the truck, accompanied by another fiery blast of air, Louise had already begun to panic. We were as close to the middle of nowhere as either of us had ever been, it was hotter than hell, and it was getting dark. Although it was only 35 miles to the next dot on the map, Beatty, Nevada, we had no idea whether this was any more of a town than Stovepipe Wells. And, from the looks of things, Beatty seemed to occupy its own niche of the middle of nowhere.

"I'm not going any further," Louise said. There was a cheery looking resort across the road from the closed ranger station, as unlikely as a mirage. It had a restaurant and bar, and industrial-sized air-conditioning units on the roof. Where they got their electricity for all this was unclear. It was like finding a self-contained life-supporting outpost on another planet.

"How much for a room for two for one night?" I asked the woman behind the desk.

"Well, sir," she replied, with a smug look. "If I *had* a room, which I don't, it would run about a hundred and fifteen dollars. That's if I had a room, which I don't." She repeated this information for her own satisfaction.

"Nothing?" I asked.

"As I have already said, sir, twice, I got nothing." She arranged a smile on her face and waited for me to leave.

"Any other places to stay around here?"

She chuckled to herself, and said, "Beatty, over in Nevada. They might have something. I wouldn't really know."

"No room," I said to Louise as I got back into the truck. "We have to go to Beatty, Nevada." She moaned.

As we pulled out of Stovepipe Wells and into the black night, Louise pressurized the air in the cab with silent panic. She stared straight ahead, her eyes focused on the dashboard, and she breathed as if every breath was her last. Her anxiety was so palpable that I became infected. "We're gonna get through this, I promise," I told her, patting her thigh. This caused her to flinch, and it interrupted the rhythm of her carefully controlled breathing. I concentrated on the tiny pools of light from our headlights, and grimly drove us further into the black void.

After a few minutes, I tried to lighten the mood. "You know, if we can't find a motel in Beatty, we can always camp in the desert." This was true. We were well provisioned for camping, and had just camped out a couple of nights before in the redwoods on the coast. She then spoke for the first time since Stovepipe Wells. She informed me that we would not be camping in the desert that night under any circumstances, even if it meant I had to drive us all the way to Las Vegas without stopping, and I'd better get her to a motel if I knew what was good for me. When she stopped talking, she retreated back into herself.

I returned my attention to the road. I hadn't reassured her, but I had myself. We'd been reacting to an emergency that hadn't happened. We had plenty of fuel and provisions. The truck was running great. We had every kind of tool we could need, including a crowbar and a shovel, and a good spare tire. Beatty was less than thirty miles away. I looked up. The sky was choked with stars, even down here, in the Valley of Death. All the tension fell away from me in an instant. As we climbed up out of the valley floor onto a higher plateau, and then crossed the Nevada line, the road ran northwest, straight as a string and level as a table. I laughed at our silliness, and my laugh piqued her curiosity.

"What's so funny?" she asked. I cheerfully explained why everything was okay and how we'd panicked for no reason. I rolled down my window and sped up to 85 miles per hour. The warm desert wind roared through the cab. Louise rolled her window down, too, and the spell was broken. "Wahoo!" I hollered out the window. Driving at high speed through the desert at night with the windows open is a great pleasure, and was just what we needed.

When we got to Beatty, we drove from motel to motel. The first four each had a No Vacancy sign glowing in the window, and with each disappointment, Louise retreated a little further back into herself. At the fifth motel, we saw a big beautiful red neon sign in the lobby window that said Vacancy. We parked right in front of the sign. The cheerfully lit lobby was fully visible behind the plate glass. A nice-looking lady sat behind the counter, typing into a computer. I got out to claim our room. We were delivered from the Valley of Death! Clean sheets, air conditioning, cable TV!

"We need a room for two for one night," I said to the nice-looking lady, and didn't bother to ask about the price.

The smile left her face and she gasped, her hand covering her mouth. "Oh, I'm so sorry. I forgot to turn on the No. I'm very sorry. We're full." She turned on the No.

I spun around to look at Louise. She looked as if someone had slapped her hard in the face, and she was looking at me. As if *I* had slapped her. The No Vacancy neon reflected across the windshield. She told me later that she could see from my expression that the last thing in the world I wanted to do was walk back out to the pickup and get into the cab with her. I turned back to the lady, who had become ugly to me–who, in fact, now looked to me like a dried up exotic dancer, too old for Vegas, expelled to Beatty, "The Gateway to Death Valley," to while away her few remaining years. "Is there anyplace else we might try?" I asked, hopelessly.

She wrinkled up her forehead as she thought about it. "Well, you might try El Portal. It's out at the edge of town."

We'd driven past El Portal as we'd entered Beatty. We'd not noticed it because it was so dark. It was the last building on the edge of town, set well back from the road with a large unlit parking lot. I parked in front of the door. The front of the building was lit only by my headlights and the doorbell button, which I pushed. I waited uncertainly, as people do when they push a doorbell they can't hear, until a light came on and the door swung open. Louise slipped out of the truck and up close behind me.

A kindly looking old man who looked as if he'd been resting for a long time said "Good evening." He beckoned us in and went through another door and re-emerged behind the counter, where he took his seat and put on his glasses. He stretched his face, which made a quick series of antic expressions and settled back into a comfortable-looking sag. He ran his finger and thumb across his improbably black pencil thin moustache, and looked at me, smiling patiently.

"Do you have any rooms?" I ventured. Louise was pressing against my back.

214

"All I got left's a couple of smoking rooms." This seemed to remind him that he could use a cigarette. He patted himself down, found a cigarette, and lit it within about two seconds.

"That'll be fine. We'll take one. How much?" I had produced my wallet and credit card. He ran it through a vintage credit card swiper.

El Portal seemed to date from the 1940s. Our room was much larger than the standard motel room of today. Everything was clean, but deeply worn. Nothing seemed to have been changed since it was built, from the smoke-stained wallpaper and drapes, to the bullfighter prints, to the bedspread and pillows, to the threadbare towels hanging by the Formica sink counter, which was worn through to the underlying wood in places and accented by cigarette-burn marks from the ages. The carpet had a path worn in it from the front door to the sink and bathroom at the opposite end, with a side-path to the bed on the left. Louise peeked in and decided to wait outside by the door while I transferred everything of value from the truck to the room. Then, clutching her own pillow from home, she tiptoed to the bed, staying on the worn path, sat down, removed her shoes and placed them carefully where her feet could slip back into them at a moment's notice. I brought her a sleeping pill and water. As soon as she'd swallowed it, she slipped under the covers fully dressed, settled her head on her pillow, pulled the covers up to her chin, and waited to be transported to the underworld.

I'd noticed a yellowed sign beside an empty postcard rack in the tiny lobby that had listed the amenities of El Portal:

*Air Conditioning *

Color TV

Pool

I changed into swimming trunks, grabbed one of the see-through towels, and crunched across the parking lot in my cowboy boots in search of the pool. It was behind the lobby building. The pool was a full eight feet deep at one end, and unlit except by starlight. I dove in and spent a relaxing half-hour swimming laps, diving and lounging in the cool water, looking up at the stars. When I got back to the room, Louise was in the underworld or pretending to be. I quickly joined her.

Las Vegas

I told that story to Joe, Laura, and Annie as we drove through Beatty and continued on toward Las Vegas.

I used to worry about Las Vegas. When every place becomes Vegas, what becomes of Vegas? Before the return of riverboat gambling, and the advent of Indian casinos all over the country, Las Vegas filled a valuable niche in American civilization. It was a biblical place—an oasis for a Christian nation, far out in the desert, where Americans went for therapeutic doses of both the pleasures and dangers of sin. With a wicked gleam in our eyes, we'd tell our closest friends where we were going. We'd drive the station wagon to the airport and leave our upright lives behind for an illicit, extra-long weekend. We felt lucky, as we surrendered ourselves to the thieves and cutthroats who ran the place, the whores and naked dancers, the card sharks and rigged roulette wheels, the cheap drinks and darker intoxicants. We felt lucky, win or lose, as we indulged in a few nights of role-play among strangers, dressed as best we could to emulate the gangsters and fleshpots waiting there to fleece and titillate us. It was great to have such a place in America, a place set aside for sin. It was right that we had to undertake a journey to get there. It was fitting that it was far out into the desert. And it was so satisfying, once we'd journeyed back home, for each of us to tell our Vegas story as our friends leaned in to hear it.

Now, Las Vegas is just like a thousand other places, only more so. This used to make me a bit sad to contemplate, but it doesn't anymore. Las Vegas has outgrown its usefulness, just as it's outgrown its desert site. It's a doomed city, and for good reasons.

Neither Joe nor Laura nor I considered ourselves "the Vegas type," and none of us had ever been there. (That's not quite true. I'd been to Las Vegas once when I was a truck driver. I'd delivered a load of tile from Tulsa to a warehouse, located in some light-industrial edge of the city. I delivered the load, had a cheap breakfast, and left. I never saw anything that told me where I was, except for a slot machine in the restaurant. And, truth be told, Louise and I had sped through Las Vegas on an expressway at high noon, after passing through the Valley of Death, but we weren't curious enough about the place to slow down.) Annie, on the other hand was intensely curious about the place, being both young and European. When we saw the sky begin to glow up ahead, as we approached the place, she leaned forward in anticipation.

Joe, on the other hand, had become alarmed. He asked me from the backseat how we could go *around* Las Vegas. The city was a dangerously concentrated distillation of everything vulgar that he despised about American culture. Coming in contact with it could be morally fatal.

"Not possible, Joe. We have to go right through the middle."

He began to moan. Once we'd passed the Bruce Woodbury Beltway, we'd figuratively passed through the gates to the city. "Don't slow down!" Joe commanded. He'd begun squirming in his seat. "In fact, speed up!"

"Where is everything?" Annie asked, craning her neck for the Las Vegas of her dreams.

Laura had caught Annie's enthusiasm and was also looking intently out the windows for Las Vegas, that is to say, for The Strip.

We passed I-15 and there it was, the great, doomed city, in all its crass defiance. It was a little after 11:00 p.m. on the Fourth of July in the city of no clocks. I'd expected fireworks. Either we were too late, or they were ongoing but swallowed up by the neon.

"I want to see!" Annie squealed.

"Close your eyes!" Joe shouted to us all, and then he became inarticulate. He began to moan. Annie and Laura opened their eyes wider.

I exited onto Las Vegas Boulevard, plunging us into the belly of the beast.

"Turn back!" Joe pleaded.

"Can't, Joe." We were in bumper-to-bumper, stop-and-go traffic, traveling down The Strip at approximately pedestrian speed. There were thousands of people, all around us, moving in throngs.

"U-turn," Joe called out. "Here's a spot! Let me have the wheel!"

As the rest of us surrendered to our astonishment in the neon wonderland, Joe grew quiet. The only way out was forward, he understood, and he surrendered also. The next time he spoke he mumbled that it was all "pretty damned amazing." Wretchedly vulgar, but amazing nonetheless.

In most American cities, motels line the beltway around the edge of town. Las Vegas is the opposite. All accommodations appear to be concentrated in the center. There may even be an ordinance against motels on the outer edges. Once we'd passed through the belly of the beast, and thereafter found ourselves excreted out the other end, we spent a frustrating half-hour searching for a place to stay. By then we were all tired from a long day of driving and the sensory overload of The Strip, so tempers flared. I was driving, and Joe and Laura, consulting competing maps, shouted contradictory instructions at me at every intersection. We searched in vain for a motel. After a couple of irrational U-turns, I pulled into a dark parking lot and stopped. "I can't do this anymore," I announced. I got out of the Rover and stood on the pavement in front of it, feeling spiky and jagged, and waited for Joe and Laura to come up with a unified escape plan.

Joe came out with his map. He spread it across the hood and showed me the plan, at which I shrugged. He took the wheel. I took his vacated seat and settled into a sullen silence. As Las Vegas receded in our mirrors, Joe instructed Annie to not look back. Her folks would never forgive him, I imagined him thinking, if he had to ship her home as a pillar of salt. I don't know about Annie, but I did look back, and as I did, I decided, in my sulkiness, that things hadn't gone that well in Vegas.

Crossing the Colorado

Somewhere along the way to Boulder City, Joe stopped at a convenience store for gas. We all got out to stretch while he filled the tank. I walked around the building, taking big steps to stretch my legs, and trying unsuccessfully to dispel my hostile feelings. I went inside. Laura was at the checkout with two bottles of water. I snatched a pack of chewing gum off the counter rack and tossed it alongside her waters just as her purchase was being rung up. My gum got caught up in her transaction, which had been my intention. Laura gave me a look but didn't say anything. When I pocketed the gum, she gave me another look. Why had I done that? I don't usually even chew gum. Neither of us spoke during this transgression. This was rude, bad behavior on my part, which I didn't understand, but couldn't seem to stop myself from doing. There would be consequences, to my bad behavior.

We found rooms in Boulder City in a run-down motel. My room had air-conditioning problems. I had a hot, restless night.

As I crossed the road, groggy and baggy-eyed, to get to a Starbucks, I encountered Laura on her way back to the motel with a cup of coffee. The sun was just coming up, loaded with the day's promises.

"'Mornin', Laura." We stopped in the middle of the road.

She smiled. "Good morning. This cool air is nice. You sleep okay?" She sipped her coffee.

"Not really. My room was hot." The desert breeze blew down the road around us, kicking up bits of paper and sandy dust.

"Too bad. You've got a long day ahead." We walked on. She seemed friendly, I thought, and I was ready to make nice with her and Joe after my sulk. I just needed a cup of coffee first.

Then There Is No Mountain

Joe was sitting in the Starbucks having coffee and a roll and leafing through a newspaper. He seemed to be examining it more than reading it. I dug around in my pockets and pulled out a handful of sticky quarters that I'd managed to accumulate. I stacked the quarters in stacks of four by the register to pay for coffee and a roll. The girl behind the counter sanitized her hands after counting them into the register and handing me my goods. I sat down with Joe.

He put the paper away. "I have some good news and some bad news," he announced.

I took the lid off my coffee, leaned into it until my nose was just above the hot, black liquid, and took a deep breath through my nose, savoring the aroma, letting the steam soften the bags under my eyes. Then I blew across the surface, rippling it, breaking up the light reflecting from the overhead lamp. Then I took two noisy sips. "Okay. What's the bad news?"

"We're driving straight through, all the way from here to Tulsa."

"We can't do that. That's twelve-hundred miles." I shook my head.

"We have to."

"But why?"

"Because once Laura and Annie get off this evening in Albuquerque, Laura's done with us. She's been paying for everything since Portland, from rooms at the Mark Hopkins to chewing gum at 7-Elevens. After Albuquerque, we're on our own."

I slumped in my seat and took a drink of coffee. I had no argument for this. I tried to change the subject. "Well, what's the good news?"

"The good news?"

"Yeah. I'm ready for the good news now."

"The good news is, is——-"

"Yes?"

"I can't remember the good news."

"Try to remember, Joe. It's important."

"Oh. I remember now. That was the good news."

"That was the good news? Jesus Christ, what's the bad news?"

"There is no bad news."

I retreated into my coffee again. I was in no condition to match wits. "Did I mention that it's twelve-hundred miles?" I asked after a while.

"Yes. One-thousand one-hundred and ninety-five, actually, according to Google maps. It's going to be great. We can do this. It's going to be—"

"Great. Right. We can't do this. I'm already tired, and I just got up. It was too hot in my room last night. I didn't sleep well at all."

"We can do this. A twelve-hundred mile run. Think about what a cool thing that is to do. You and me, just like Kerouac and Cassady. It's cool, man! Come on!"

"Joe, we're not exactly half our age."

He scoffed at this nonsensical comment. "Agreed. We're not even approximately half our age. We'd better get started."

We carried our coffees back across the road. Boulder City seemed to be on the verge of waking up. A couple of cars rounded a corner. A kid pedaled along on a bicycle. I didn't like any of it. Boulder City was originally built as a work camp for construction of the iconic Boulder Dam, later renamed

Hoover Dam. These days, its gauche lakeview faux-mansions, with their xe-riscaped grounds, tacky statuary, and swimming pools of stolen water make Boulder City look like a millionaire pornographer's wet dream of a great place to raise his children.

Crossing Hoover Dam has never been a casual undertaking. The first time I'd crossed it was in a tractor-trailer just before dawn fifteen years ear-lier. I'd come switchbacking down into the Colorado River gorge from the Arizona side. Rounding the last bend, I saw the dam's Buck Rogers-style tur-rets rising from the water. I saw the dam's deep curve pushing back against the lake. I saw an ambulance crew and tow-truck crew standing by in their idling vehicles. When I crept across the narrow two-lane road atop the dam in that big rig, I was sitting high above the deck, and far enough above the low guardrail that I couldn't see it, which made me feel dizzy. The gorge dropped down on my left to a hidden dark depth. High-voltage transmission towers leaned out toward each other over the gorge at crazy angles. On the other side the smooth water of Lake Mead had just begun to reflect a bit of soft light back at the sky. At the other end of the dam were another idling ambulance, tow truck, and even a police station. Pulling my load up out of the gorge was steep and slow going.

Since 9/11, Hoover Dam has been considered by Homeland Security a juicy target for terrorists. It's not hard to imagine why. The dam is a focal point of power in the West. The lake behind it is a crucial source of electricity and water for western cities and agriculture, and the dam is the only Colorado River crossing for many miles in either direction. Consequently, the drama of crossing has now been dulled by the tedium of various road blocks, vehicle checks, and the showing of papers to armed men. Once the authorities had run mirrors under the Rover and cleared us to cross, we also had to negotiate construction traffic for the magnificent bridge being built to span the gorge just downstream from the dam. When they finish the bridge, the dam will be closed to vehicular traffic.

On the Arizona side we parked to take pictures. The bridge under construction was as impressive to me as the dam. It will cross the gorge at a higher level. When I'd seen it two years earlier, in its beginning phase, I'd

224

assumed they'd span the gorge with a suspension bridge. Instead they'd had the audacity to build a soaring concrete arch over the gorge. By the time Joe and I stood there studying it, two concrete arcs had been raised from opposite cliffs, straining over the gorge to meet at their highpoint in the center, over the thrashing river a thousand feet below. There remained only a narrow gap left between the arcs. Twin crews crawled around on each point. From where we stood, they appeared to be within easy shouting distance of each other. Welders straddled I-beams with nothing beneath their boots but air and hell.

The overlook where we stood wasn't built for viewing the bridge. It was to view Hoover Dam and Lake Mead. By studying the dwindling lake's bathtub rings on the surrounding cliffs, Joe calculated that the water level had dropped by about 80 feet from its normal level. Nature was slowly but surely taking back the Colorado River gorge, and in the process, doing what no mad bomber could: ultimately cutting off water and electricity to much of the West, thereby dooming thirsty desert cities. Most especially Las Vegas, which had grown far beyond any sustainable scale. This thrilled Joe's inner anarchist, no doubt (and mine as well, I must admit). He looked over the disappearing reservoir, nodding slightly to himself, his eyes hidden by the reflection on his glasses.

On the desert road to Flagstaff, we saw freshly painted "Land For Sale" signs, offering parcels indistinguishable from the rest of the landscape. These were being offered in anticipation of the expected influx of traffic from I-40 to Las Vegas, once the bridge is completed. Will it be a bridge to nowhere, in the end? I wondered.

Flagstaff

Joe, Laura, and I had been to Flagstaff the year before, along with Arne, a lanky, good-natured German exchange student who'd been spending the school year with Joe and Laura. We'd come there to climb Humphrey's Peak. Humphrey's is in the San Francisco range of extinct volcanoes, and, at 12,633 feet, is the highest point in Arizona. It creates a scenic backdrop just north of Flagstaff. It had been the first day of spring, so there were still several feet of snow covering most of the mountainside. We'd driven up to the ski lodge, donned snowshoes and backpacks, and started climbing. Since the trail and its markers were buried in the snow, we made our way up the steep slope through the pine forest by dead reckoning. Above the treeline, and a few hundred feet below the rim, our wayward path took us by the wreckage of a B-24 bomber that had crashed into the mountainside during a night training mission on September 15, 1944. We'd read about the crash and wreckage in a guidebook. It was a well-known landmark on the mountain. However, we hadn't expected to come across it, and when we did, we realized we were about a quarter of a mile north of where we thought we were. From there to the rim was a difficult scrabble over loose scree and patches of snow. Humphrey's is a relatively isolated peak, so the view from the rim seemed to stretch out forever in all directions. We could see the Grand Canyon off to the north.

After catching our breath, we discussed our situation, and made a difficult decision. We only had about two hours of daylight left, and we estimated that the summit was still about a twenty-minute hike along the rim. If we estimated it at twenty minutes there, then it would probably turn out to be thirty, then another thirty minutes back to where we stood. If we bagged the summit, we'd not be able to make it back to the ski lodge before dark. So, three of us decided that we had to turn back. Arne tried hard to convince us that we could do it, and became angry when we refused to budge. He fumed as the rest of us enjoyed the view for a few minutes. On the way down, he plunged ahead, his snowshoed legs flailing away.

I've now climbed three state highpoints with Joe and Laura, and one with Joe. I've only reached the summit on one of them. There are people who make it a life-goal to climb to the highpoint of every state, and they are known as highpointers. I've become a highpointer in a different sense, having climbed *high* enough in New Mexico, Arizona, and Washington *point* to the summit. In fairness, I have reached the highpoints of Indiana and Kansas, and also, my favorite, Black Mesa, a lonely, haunting, and beautiful place in the extreme northwest corner of the Oklahoma panhandle, which tops out at 4,973 feet.

On this trip, around midday we arrived in Flagstaff, a pleasant, prosperous western city of about 60,000. We parked near a farmer's market and walked five blocks to the downtown business district to find a place for lunch. Once we were in the business district, Joe and Laura were unable to cooperate in deciding where to eat. "How about that place?" Joe would suggest. "No," Laura would reply. "We could try there," Laura would venture. "That doesn't look good to me," Joe would reply. "Let's eat there." "No, Joe." And so on. These exchanges became heated. Annie and I, as their wards, tagged uselessly along behind them as we all lurched forward, stalled, made U-turns. Then they changed tactics, which brought things to a standstill on the sidewalk. "You decide." "No, you." "I'll eat wherever you say." "No, Joe. Just pick where you want us to eat. Whatever." "No, Laura. You pick. I don't care anymore." And so on. Annie and I glanced at each other and studied the shop windows as this went on. They turned to me. "Rich, will you pick out a place to eat, please?" Laura requested.

As a matter of fact, there was a diner a half-block away where we'd had a good breakfast the year before. Joe and Laura trailed unhappily behind me. They seemed to have finally found an eating place they could agree on, in that neither of them liked my choice. Annie was as inscrutable as ever. We settled into a booth. Joe and Laura sat across from Annie and me. They each stared straight ahead, not speaking. The waitress distributed menus and waters, which Joe and Laura ignored. When she returned for our orders, Laura said, "Nothing for me." Joe just shook his head. Annie, taking her cue from them, said, "I'll have nothing, please." I ordered a club sandwich. We sat there in silence for three or four minutes, during which time I became angry.

I stood, went to the cash register, and told the cashier that I'd ordered a club sandwich, and that I would like them to make it to go, and that I'd like to go ahead and pay for it. The cash register accepted my debit card–reluctantly, it seemed to me. I could deal with the overdraft charges later.

After paying, I went outside, secretly amused, in a bitter kind of way, that my three companions, who'd refused to order anything, were now silently holding up commerce during the lunch rush. In the plaza across the street, some local Indians in full regalia were putting on a show for the tourists. I strolled over to watch for a while. When I went back to the diner to get my sandwich, Joe, Laura, and Annie had left. I ate my sandwich in the sunny plaza. At 7,000 feet elevation, the summer air in Flagstaff was light and fresh. I began to feel much better. The air energized me and improved my mood. I saw Annie window shopping alone near the diner. I caught up with her and led her back across the street, so she could see the dancers. She watched with intense interest. At this point in the performance, the dancers were all young men. "Where's your camera?" I asked. "Oh, I left it in the Land Rover," she replied disappointedly. "So, let's go get it." "No, it's too far." "It's not too far." "Are you sure?" "Yes. You have to photograph this, Annie." Her fraulein friends back in Germany would swoon with envy when she showed them her pictures of these brawny exotics in feathers and skins. "Come on," I urged. She happily fell into step beside me. We hiked back to our parking spot with long, quick steps, stretching our legs and working our lungs. It was invigorating, and expelled all the frustrations from earlier. When we got back, the dancers were still performing. Annie snapped happily away. Joe walked up. "Have you seen Laura?" he asked. "No." He walked on. Laura walked up. "Have you seen Joe?" "He went thataway." She walked on.

Before long, everyone found everyone, and we all strolled companionably back to the Rover together. All the tensions of lunch, and of the night before, seemed to have wisped away. But there was a deeper tension still in me. Surely Laura wasn't really going to abandon us out there on the highway, so far from home. Surely Joe didn't really believe we could drive straight through.

Then There Is No Mountain

Once we were on I-40 eastbound, I summoned the courage to try to reason with Laura. "Laura," I said, leaning forward from the backseat. Joe was driving, Laura sitting shotgun.

"Yes, Rich?" she replied, turning around to face me.

I could tell instantly from the tone of her voice that she knew exactly what I had been about to say. The look on her face confirmed it. How did she know? It unnerved me. "Would you like a stick of gum?" I offered. I held the pack out to her.

"Why, yes, Rich. Thank you!" She took two. I watched her unwrap them and stick them both in her mouth. She noticed me watching her, and I was still leaning forward. "Is there something else?" she asked innocently.

"Well. Yes, actually. I, I, did I ever tell you about the time I nearly killed myself and another driver on I-40 in Knoxville?"

"Don't think so. Joe, have you heard this one?"

"Probably, but go ahead."

Trucker Tales

I was hired by J. B. Hunt Trucking upon graduating from truck driving school in Drumright, Oklahoma. I believe it was about 1994. Hunt put me with an experienced driver for a few weeks to teach me those things about truck driving that couldn't be taught in school. An important fact about truck driving is that if the wheels aren't rolling, nobody is making any money. Not the customer, not the trucking company, and not the driver. So a good driver is able to lie down in the sleeper and fall asleep anytime, day or night. Rest opportunities must be taken as they come, which is pretty random. Regular hours are a luxury not available to a long haul driver. After a couple of weeks, my trainer began trying to train me for this by making me drive the late, late hours, while he slept his turn in the sleeper. About three o'clock one morning, I was driving on I-40 past the city center of Knoxville, Tennessee, while my trainer slept in the sleeper. I'd been fighting fatigue, but I knew I had to "learn" this, and figured I could get us past Knoxville before I would need to wake him and give up the wheel.

I was driving at highway speed on the expressway, and then I was driving down an off-ramp toward a traffic light at the bottom. Still at highway speed. Bewildered, I slammed on the brakes. Sixty-five feet long, eighty-thousand pounds, sixty miles an hour. When the brakes caught, it rolled my trainer right out of the sleeper. He bolted upright next to me. "What's goin' on?" he yelled in my ear. "I don't know!" I yelled back, standing on the brake. A cloud of blue smoke swirled around us as it caught up with the slowing truck. When I got us stopped, we were about six feet out into the deserted, three a.m. intersection under a red light. We looked at each other as the cloud of smoke sailed past the cab. I'm sure my eyes were as wide as his. He looked unfamiliar to me. He wore an expression I'd never seen, and he hadn't put on his thick glasses. "What happened?" he demanded, although he knew the answer. "I don't know. We were on the highway and then—" I shrugged. "You fell asleep." "I don't understand. I was just driving along." I couldn't figure out anything else to say. I had fallen asleep. That was undeniable.

"That's unfortunate. How will you survive while Annie and I are put-tin' on the Ritz at the Santa Fe Opera?" She smacked her chewing gum. "How did you end up broke, anyway?"

"Well, you see, Joe's broke because he covered most of my expenses on the drive out, and also the cost of the climb."

"Uh huh. Then how did you get broke?"

"Well, you see, I covered his expenses after he got broke." It was all perfectly logical.

When she stopped laughing, she suggested that a couple of mountain men like us could pull over and camp if we got tired. She was right, of course, and she'd been extremely generous, even considering my bad behavior the night before, but none of that mattered, because we'd both begun to enjoy the repartee.

"We don't have any camping gear," I countered. "Just climbing gear."

"Then I guess one of you will have to sleep while the other one drives."

"Can't. I have a condition."

"Oh, come on. You can do better than that."

"I'm serious. I can't sleep in a moving vehicle unless I'm driving. I don't trust anyone else to drive while I'm sleeping. That's why I'm not sleeping now, even though I'm exhausted after tossing and turning in the heat all last night."

"That is a problem. But it's not my problem."

"Joe, will you reason with her?"

"Too late, Rich. She already reasoned with me first. Give it up, bro. This is not like you. We're driving straight through. We don't need her." He turned to her. "We don't need you." They made playful faces at each other.

"Annie, will you reason with her? She listens to you." I turned to Annie beside me. She still had her earbuds in and was still looking out the window. She had no idea I'd spoken to her.

"Tell us another truck-driving story," Laura suggested. "If it's good enough, I might change my mind. Just don't count on it."

I took a deep breath, and summoned up a story. "Okay. Did I ever tell you about how bad forty-thousand pounds of fresh chicken meat smells?"

I pulled into a chicken processing plant somewhere in Alabama to pick up forty-thousand pounds of fresh chicken meat for delivery to L.A. This place was hell for chickens. A large complex of buildings, and all day and night a steady stream of trucks delivering live chickens in one end, and another steady stream of trucks pulling away from the other end filled with fresh—very fresh—chicken meat. It was staffed by Mexicans wearing hairnets and white guys wearing hardhats.

When I was a kid, and up into my young adulthood, the South had had its own smell for me. An intoxicating smell of humid decay laced with orange peels and coffee grounds. I'd always loved that smell, which I also associated with my sweet, fat grandmother and her Ozark log cabin. It's been a long time since the South has smelled that way to me. I won't describe how it smelled while I waited for my load that night in Alabama. I pulled out with the load secured and the reefer set, and headed to L.A.

When I arrived in L.A. three days later, I delivered the meat to a McDonald's facility where they would process the fresh-never-frozen meat into McNuggets and the like. The reefer had kept the load just a couple of degrees above freezing, but it didn't matter how well refrigerated it was, forty-thousand pounds of meat confined into a tightly sealed container for three days was going to leave a powerful stench behind. When I pulled away empty from the dock and walked back to close the trailer doors, I ran into the smell like running into a brick wall. It brought tears to my eyes, and nearly knocked me down.

I got the doors closed, breathing into my shirtsleeve, and headed out to a truckstop in Fontana, where I paid a trailerwash vendor to clean it out. They spent an hour hosing it out with high pressure hoses and strong detergents, and rinsing it down. I parked overnight at the truckstop with the trailer doors open so it could air out.

Next day I got dispatched to a nearby Otis Spunkmeyer cookie-dough factory to get a load of dough for delivery to Omaha. I pulled up to the dock, and a dockworker came driving up with the first forklift load of dough, pulled into the trailer, and backed right out immediately. He backed up, about fifteen feet away from the trailer, and called out to me, "What's that awful smell in there?"

It didn't seem that bad to me. "Chicken meat!" I called back. "Heck, you should've smelled it before!" I added.

A supervisor came over, took a whiff, made a face, and said, "Mister, get this trailer away from our dock. This dough'll soak up that smell like a sponge. "

"But—"

"No buts, get the hell outta here!"

I pulled away from the dock, parked as far away as I could on their property, and called my dispatcher. He'd been in the game for a while, and he knew just what to do. "Here's what I want you to do. Drop the trailer, bobtail to a grocery store, and buy two big cans of coffee. Folger's Aromatic Blend, if you can find it. Spread those coffee grounds all over the floor of that trailer, seal it up, and run the reefer all night to circulate the air. By morning it ought to be okay."

Feeling a little giddy with permission to bobtail, I found a store, bought the coffee, and did as I was told. Then I bobtailed over to Hawthorne, hometown of the Beach Boys. I walked around on the beach for a little while, and went out to dinner at a vegetarian place. The food was awful. They had, over the kitchen doorway, a framed photo of Paul McCartney posing with the owner.

Next morning, I swept the coffee out of the trailer and pulled back up to the dock. When the same supervisor saw that it was me, he walked over, prepared to run me off again if necessary.

"I think you're gonna like this!" I said with a proud smile. "Go ahead. Take a big whiff."

He stuck his head inside the trailer and took a deep breath. "Nice!" he smiled. "Real nice!" A half-hour later, as I signed for the load of dough, he said, "Now, we need you to hurry, driver. They're almost out of cookies in Omaha. Okay?"

"I will fly like the wind," I replied. "For the children. The children of Omaha."

Laura's response to this story was to ask Joe if he'd brought along any audio books.

"But wait!" I interjected before he could reply. "Let me tell you about the time I got into a fight in Madison, Wisconsin!"

I was just passing through Madison, but I had some slack time, and I'd always been curious about the city, remembering the university there as a hotbed of radicalism in the Sixties. I parked in the back row of a truckstop north of town that evening, caught up my logbook, waved off a truckstop whore, unhooked from my trailer, and bobtailed into town.

I parked about three or four dark, deserted blocks from the Capitol building, and hiked past the Capitol to the thriving business district skirting the University of Wisconsin campus. After weeks of highway isolation I walked in love through the crowds of students, all those laughing pretty girls, and those happy loud boys, out for supper and an evening's carouse. I claimed a table for two in a crowded bistro, where I ate a sandwich, and drank deeply from the loud music of their voices, above the clatter and clink. Whenever anyone brushed against me in the crowded space, my nerves stood on end for more. I was thirsty for human contact, but couldn't reach out, couldn't look anyone in the eye. Too many weeks on the highway. Back on the street I strolled the crowded sidewalks, aching for every shapely girl twisting past, and content just to ache, my pulse racing, my head spinning.

It was a pleasantly warm night, and a used bookstore with an open door drew me in. I'd been looking for a copy *of* "The Log Of A Cowboy" by Andy Adams, and, after a few satisfying minutes browsing the shelves, I found an early-edition copy in like-new condition, reasonably priced. Before purchasing it, I sat down in a tattered wingback chair, near the store's big front window, to leaf through it.

Three older gentlemen were seated near me, two on a worn sofa and one in a chair like mine. They were swapping tales of their glory days as professors in the heated Sixties, when they'd "taken it to the streets" (following a safe distance behind their students, I soon gathered). They were like old soldiers everywhere, except that, being professors, they spoke more loudly than most, as they tried to outdo each other's tales of derring-do. The battles they recounted so fondly, it seemed to me, had mostly to do with intramural turf wars with less radical administrators during the protracted aftermath of their beloved students' actual streetfights. They spoke beyond each other to the room at large, which soon annoyed me. It was time for me to go settle into my truck and read about the longest cattle drive ever attempted.

Book in hand, I hiked back past the Capitol, beyond which the sidewalks were deserted, and the buildings locked and dark. I saw another lone male figure walking toward me a block and a half up ahead. I didn't know why, but I knew I didn't want to pass this stranger, so I casually angled across the street. He did the same thing. I don't know how I knew, but I knew this meant trouble. When we arrived simultaneously at the sidewalk on the other side, we were about a half block apart. When we reached each other he lunged at me, grasping for my throat, and growled, "I'm gonna kill you."

Then There Is No Mountain

Before I could think to do it, I'd already forced both of my arms upward and outward between his, wedging his striving fingers away from my throat. Then, I drew my arm back, and with every ounce of strength in me, I jammed the spine of my book into his adam's apple. The force of the blow should have collapsed his windpipe. But instead of falling to the ground and choking to death at my feet, he staggered backwards three steps. Then, for the first time, he actually looked at me. What he saw, there under our shared streetlight, was a man ready to fight.

I was facing him squarely, my hands down but away from my sides, and my right hand clutching the book, which he knew I knew how to use. I was staring deeply into his eyes. I didn't move as I waited for him to move toward me. I wasn't afraid. I don't know why.

After about ten seconds, he said, hoarsely, "You might be bigger than me, but I could still whip your ass." This was nonsense because he was about six inches taller and thirty pounds heavier than me. I made no response. We stared at each other for a few more seconds.

I turned my back on him and walked deliberately away, neither fast nor slow, not looking back. Although I appeared to have forgotten about him, I was listening intensely for any sound of him following, but I heard only my own bootsteps. I hadn't spoken a word during our violent encounter. Back in the safety of my locked cab, I discovered that I'd hit him so hard that it had cracked the book's front cover from top to bottom. Evidently my aim had been off, and the blow that was meant to kill had glanced first off his chin, which had absorbed most of the impact. That chin had broken my book, forever now demoted from like-new condition. On the other hand, it's now a book with two stories instead of one.

"That's a pretty good story," Joe said, after due consideration.

Laura nodded her head in agreement.

"So--?" I ventured.

238

"No."

"Aw, man! I'm working so hard here!"

"Hey, Rich," Joe said into his rearview mirror. We locked eyes. "Surrender, bro".

I looked out the window for a good long while. "Okay, then. I surrender," I announced, finally.

"Good man!" Joe replied. We grinned at each other in the mirror.

Interstate 40 had been laid alongside, and on top of, the old Route 66. The towns and attractions of that legendary old road had streamed past us as I'd told my stories: Meteor Crater, Winslow, Jackrabbit Trading Post, Holbrook, The Petrified Forest, The Painted Desert, Gallup, Grants, and all the Indian Trading Posts along the way. Since Route 66 -also known as The Mother Road, The Main Street of America, and The Will Rogers Highway- was decommissioned on June 27, 1985, it has, after a burst of renewed interest triggered by the decommission, returned to its slow fade from the collective American memory. It was, for a long time, a conduit for our dreams of a somehow better future, and then for our dreams of a somehow better past. The number of those who remember its cultural significance grows smaller all the time, and the number of those who still pine for it grows smaller still. Over the years, I've driven every mile of it, from the steps of the Art Institute of Chicago to the Santa Monica Pier.

My brother Mike was the founding president of the Oklahoma Chapter of the Route 66 Association, soon after decommission. Mike and I used to take day-trips along the old Oklahoma "alignments," photographing falling-down motels and gas stations, fading painted signs on old brick walls, fissured white lines on orphaned sections of aged asphalt. We were intensely nostalgic for an America we never really knew. But that nostalgia has faded in me, as it has in the culture more generally. In Tulsa, in the summer, we still see occasional pilgrims passing through along the old route. Motorcyclists, RVs, hitchhikers, and long-haul bicyclists, but not as many as there used to be.

We four rode in silence for miles. Then Joe turned around in the driver's seat and, with gestures, communicated to Annie to take out her earbuds, which she did. "Hey, Rich," he said to me, "why don't you tell Annie about the time you found Satan's skull."

Annie looked at me. "Satan's skull?" she asked, to make sure she'd heard it right.

I nodded gravely.

"But where?"

"West Texas. Where else?"

"Are you putting me on, Rich?"

I loved the way she said that with her German accent.

"I wouldn't do that, Annie. Not about something this important."

I forget what I was hauling, but I was heading west out of Houston pulling a reefer on I-10. I passed through San Antonio, then Kerrville, then out onto the Edwards Plateau, the Texas outback, hundreds of miles of sparsely populated high scrubland. There were a few thin clouds in the late afternoon sky, softening the sun as it centered itself in my windshield. Traffic had thinned to nothing. From where I sat, except for the highway, there were few visible signs of man. A line of white limestone cliffs rose to the right, running along about a half-mile or so from the roadway. Near the top of the highest one, I saw a cave. It struck me as an obvious place for aboriginal shelter. By a strange coincidence, an exit ramp presented itself right up ahead. Without quite *deciding* to, I braked and pulled off. At the top of the ramp was an overpass to the left, an onramp straight ahead, and a locked gate to the right. Beyond the gate was an overgrown two-track leading unconvincingly out into the scrub. I shut the engine off, took a long drink of water, stepped down out of the cab, locked it, and climbed the gate. I was hiking within two minutes of having seen the cave. The sound of the reefer motor quickly faded away behind me as I crunched across the loose gravel and sand.

It felt good to walk in strange country. Unfamiliar birds flitted and called out among brushy plants and flowers whose names I didn't know. I hiked uphill, following the drainage patterns. A few sheep scrambled away from my approach. They seemed as wild as antelope. As the sides of the butte steepened, every step up made the horizon jump back another ten miles. After about a thirty-minute hike I got to the cave, just under the top ridge line of the butte. I was panting slightly, my muscles tingled, and I felt alive to every moment. The cave cut back about ten feet into the cliff face and had a ceiling averaging about seven-to-eight feet. The view to the south looked like forever, with little discernible variation in the terrain or cover. Interstate 10 sliced across the land out there from horizon to horizon a hundred and fifty feet wide, and I could not see a trace of it. Strange to know that it was so easily hidden out there, half a mile away. The cave floor had been excavated. An abandoned archaeologist's screen lay against one of the sifted dirt piles. After seeing that, I didn't expect to find anything, but I poked around anyway. There were lots of flint shards, but no arrowheads or potsherds. At eyelevel on the cave wall, I found the archaeologist's signatures. Four men had signed the wall in pencil, and dated it April 4, 1947.

As a trucker, I spent most of my time moving fast, but for a few minutes I sat there on a boulder, looking out to the south, as though from my front step, joining the land in its stillness. The sun, though, edged closer to the horizon all the time. A rubble-filled crease extended down the cliff face below the cave. I worked my way down the crease, slipping on the loose scree, watching for rattlesnakes and artifacts. About halfway down, I found an arrowhead, fine edged, lustrous, and pale gray. I admired it in the failing light. From the moment that I held it in my hand, it joined the distance between me and the last man to hold it in his hand. It had flown who knows how far from him to me. Who was he? Was that a question he would have asked of himself? What world did he live in? I put it in my jeans pocket. The sun lay against the horizon. What world did *I* live in?

Then There Is No Mountain

I clambered on down the cliff and skirted my way along the base, back to a point near where I'd begun climbing earlier. It was the time of day when color begins to drain, and shadows spill out of their containers and run together over the ground. I found a narrow dry streambed to walk in. It was easier than pushing through the brush and cactus, but it twisted every which way, and deepened until the surrounding ground level was at my chin, giving me a rabbits-eye view of things. The light had flattened by the time I climbed out of the streambed. All birds had silenced and gone to roost. No leaf stirred. Like the intruder that I was, I placed each step with care, quieting my footfalls. Finding a rhythm, I slipped through the mesquite like a ghost, hyper-alert with all my senses. I came out of the thicket to the edge of a clearing and stopped cold before I quite knew why.

I held my breath, and stood frozen in place, as I took in what I saw. The clearing was round, and about thirty feet across. In the center, facing me, was a human skull. But something wasn't right. A quick gust shivered through the brush. Protruding out of the corners of the skull's forehead were two horns, each about three inches long. The skull of Satan! I might have fled, but I didn't. Instead I rushed *to* it, compelled by I don't know what. When I knelt and picked it up, a little black snake, exposed, raced away, causing me to leap backwards two full steps with the horned skull in my hands. Was Satan dead at last? I wondered as I raised his skull and gazed into those gaping black eyeholes.

And then I began laugh. I laughed loud and long, a brazen, careless insult to the hushed world. I laughed at the joke, and the joke was on me. What I held in my hand, reason assured me, was the skull of a young ram with the snout missing, which flattened it to an uncanny resemblance to a human, or a devil. I tossed it aside and walked on toward the highway and my waiting truck, inconsiderately thrashing and crunching along, erupting now and again into short bouts of laughter. By the time I heard the thrumming of my reefer motor to guide me home, it had grown dark around me. I settled into the cab, fired up the diesel, and sat smiling for a minute in the multicolored glow of the dashlights before I slipped it into gear and headed west.

Annie punched me in the shoulder. "You were putting me on! A ram's head."

"You should've seen it, Annie. Scared me half to death."

"Yah? I would love to find an arrowhead."

"I'll have to show you my collection sometime before you head back to Europe."

What was most frightening was that there had been no discontinuity in my experience. The highway had curved to the left, and I'd continued driving straight, onto a fortunately placed off-ramp as I slept for a second, or two, or three, or maybe longer. When I awoke to my new situation, there had been a seamless fitting of my perception back to the moment before I'd fallen asleep. I was driving along the highway, which *became* an off-ramp with a traffic light straight ahead. "Get out of the driver's seat," he commanded. "Heck, I'm awake now!" I joked feebly, forcing a grin. Neither of us laughed. He routed me out of the driver's seat, we got our bearings, and he soon got us back onto the highway. After a few minutes, I stepped into the sleeper, pulled the curtain, and lay down in the pitch blackness. I was rocked gently in my bunk, and the low rumble of the road hummed an old lullaby, as he took us up into the mountains.

After I'd told this story, Joe and Laura stared silently out the windshield for a few moments. Annie watched me. I waited just long enough and added, "Of course, there's a moral to the story, which is that you're a danger to yourself and others if you push yourself too hard out here on this old Interstate 40."

Joe, at the wheel, cackled. Annie put in her earbuds and looked out the window at the drab eastern Arizona desert.

Laura continued to stare out at the road. "What's your point, Rich?" she asked after a pause.

"Is it true we can't stay in a motel in Albuquerque, get some rest?"

She turned around and said, "Not true at all. You boys should stay wherever you want. Be my—oops, I almost said 'Be my guest' -but that would have been wrong. Stay where you like, just don't be my guest."

"But we're broke, Joe and me."

Venus, Oppenheimer, and Me

Just before Thoreau, New Mexico, we passed back over the Continental Divide. We were back "east," so to speak, for the first time since Wyoming. Mount Taylor dominated the view for miles and miles. We drove through its old lava flows around Grants. Just about supper time, Sandia Peak came into view ahead of us, and we dropped down into the Rio Grande Valley and the city of Albuquerque.

We met a friend of Joe and Laura's in Albuquerque for supper at a place called The Flying Star. We ate in the courtyard in the shade of tall cottonwoods, which sounded like rushing water as they whispered against each other. After a relaxing meal, Laura picked up the check one last time, and then we transferred her and Annie's baggage to their friend's car, said goodbye, and parted company.

Joe and I got back on I-40 and continued east. Just two guys on the highway, unencumbered by women or children. Or money. Our only resources were a Conoco credit card and some accumulated small change. We'd been on the move ever since Boulder City, 550 miles back down the road, and we weren't even halfway to Tulsa. We pulled up out of the valley, passed Sandia Peak, and fixed our minds on our distant destination. We passed Moriarty, Santa Rosa, Montoya, and Tucumcari. Anglo, Hispanic, and Indian—that's New Mexico.

As we passed the intersection with U.S. Highway 54, at Santa Rosa, I was reminded of the time I saw my shadow cast by Venus. "Joe, did I ever tell you about the time I camped at Three Rivers for four nights?" I asked.

"Yes."

"Fifty Four South takes you there from here. Did I tell you how strange the petroglyphs are at Three Rivers?"

Then There Is No Mountain

"I saw the pictures. Strange."

"I don't think any of us will ever really understand them."

"Goes without saying, Rich."

"I didn't camp at the glyphs, though. I camped a few miles east, at the end of the road. There's a small Forest Service campground there. It was in March, so there were only a couple of other campers. I wasn't there to make friends, and neither were they. Did I tell you that I didn't speak for four days?"

"Yes. That must have been nice."

"You have no idea."

"Hm."

"Did I tell you about the place names around there?"

"I think so."

"The campground is up on the west flank of Sierra Blanca, a couple of thousand feet above the desert floor to the west, so you have a long view. The sunsets alone were enough to strike you mute. You could see the black lava of Mal Pais, and the low silhouettes of the Oscuro Range further on."

"Mal Pais. Oscuro."

"Si. And just beyond the Oscuros, Jornada del Meurto."

"The Journey of Death."

"Yes. And did I tell you what is tucked into the back side of Oscuro Peak?"

"Truth or Consequences?"

"Trinity."

"I knew that."

"Yes?"

"Yes. I heard it from you. 'I am become Death, the Destroyer of Worlds.'"

"Krishna?"

"Oppenheimer."

"I knew that. So anyway, Joe, when they're not shooting off atomic bombs, it's dark out there. Damned dark. So, there I was, sitting on my picnic table looking west. The sun had gone down, and I had watched the last of its light drain from the sky, and the stars had begun to thicken. I was struck by how bright Venus was, hanging low in the western sky, following the sun by a couple of hours. My fire had died down to coals, so I walked over to add some wood and was struck by how well I could see. I could see my hands, my boots, my truck. I could see the dusty road beyond the camp, and I could see the shrubs and trees beyond that. All just by starlight."

"Then what happened?"

"I realized that I could see not just the forms of things, but also their shadows, and there was a direction to the shadows."

"But starlight is directionless. How can that be?"

"Are you helping me, Joe?"

"Someone has to."

Then There Is No Mountain

"So, it hit me all of a sudden. If there's no moon and no sun, and no manmade lights, what light could be casting everything's shadows? Could it be? I looked up at Venus, shining like a diamond. I walked over to the perimeter road, which was pale dust, and stood there with my back to Venus. I thought I could see a vague, smudgy shadow form, but it was so close to the edge of perception I couldn't be sure. So I lifted my right leg and swung it around a little bit."

"That's what it's all about."

"Shut up. So anyway, sure enough, my shadow moved with me. I was seeing my shadow cast by Venus."

"Freakin' awesome. What were you smoking?"

"I'm telling you I saw it."

"Were you smoking *anything?*"

"That is so beside the point."

"Is it?"

"Yes! Go there, skeptic! Next March. I dare you. Your shadow will be waiting."

"Maybe I will."

We could see lightning up ahead. Somewhere out on the Llano Estacado, around San Jon, after dark, we drove through a lengthy rainstorm, playing cat-and-mouse with it into the Texas Panhandle. By the time we drove past the Cadillac Ranch and into Amarillo, we were out of the rain, but we were road-weary. We stopped at a convenience store for water, coffee, and a good parking lot stretch. Back in the Rover, we each took an Adderall, because one of us has a prescription, chasing it with foul coffee, and got back on the highway.

248

Richard Higgs

"Hey, isn't that Pantex plant out here somewhere?" Joe asked, as the lights of Amarillo diminished behind us.

"Yeah, I think you're right. Somewhere out there just to our north." The Pantex plant, a few miles northeast of Amarillo, is one of the sites where the U.S. disarms nuclear missiles, to comply with our START treaty obligations. We looked out at the blackness. I suppose we expected to see a bright glow on the horizon, but we just saw blackness, punctuated by a few distant ranch pole lights.

Driving All Night

In the endless conversations that followed, I told Joe the story of the song, "Louie, Louie," the only song, as far as we know, to have been investigated by the FBI. It had been written in the mid 1950s by Richard Berry, an inoffensive ditty about a Caribbean sailor eager to get back to shore, to his love. It became a regional hit in the Northwest, the kind of song garage-band boys liked to play at school dances. One such band in Portland, Oregon, The Kingsmen, recorded a version of "Louie, Louie" in a one-take session at a local radio station and pressed a few copies to sell at their gigs. The lyrics, as sung by The Kingsmen's Jack Ely, were indecipherable. The record also included a slapdash guitar solo, and a false start by the singer, after the solo, which the drummer dutifully drowned out. When a copy came into the possession of a popular disc jockey in New York, he featured it on his weekly "worst record of the week" segment. It caused a teen sensation. They loved it! Soon, it was a surprise hit across the nation. When parents heard it, they went a little nuts. They couldn't comprehend how anyone could like such a raw, dumb, indecipherable recording. There must be something subversive going on! There has to be some kind of message in those lyrics that only teens can understand. Since it was rock and roll, it must be something *lewd and lascivious*. Grown-ups' paranoid and prurient obsession with the lyrics to The Kingsmens' "Louie, Louie" culminated in an investigation by the FBI. Imagine serious men in dark-blue suits wearing complicated headphones, hunched over a hi-fi that's been specially rigged to play the 45 rpm record of "Louie, Louie" at all possible speeds. Their faces grimace in concentration and outright pain. The FBI's final report on "Louie, Louie" was summed up in four words: *"Unintelligible at any speed."* The sensation became rock and roll legend. Don Preston, of the Mothers of Invention, once played the opening riff to "Louie Louie" on the mighty pipe organ at the Royal Albert Hall in London during a Mothers concert in 1969. You can hear it on "Uncle Meat." The song has been recorded many times by many groups over the decades. One hopes that Berry has lived comfortably off of the royalties.

Then There Is No Mountain

This conversation came up because Joe and I were listening to oldies radio as we drove through the night, east of Amarillo, paced by a hard white chip of moon. About ten minutes after my "Louie, Louie" disquisition, we heard its opening chords, which lit up our Adderall-infused faces with glee. We spent the next two minutes and thirty-eight seconds improvising dirty lyrics at the tops of our voices.

When we crossed the Oklahoma line, still well before dawn, I let out a long sigh of relief. Almost home. Those were Oklahoma stars above us now. Erick, Sayre, Elk City, Clinton, and Weatherford floated by. At Oklahoma City, we stopped for one last stretch and a cup of convenience-store coffee. The sky was growing light as we accelerated onto the Will Rogers Turnpike with Tulsa waiting just a hundred miles away. I'd traveled that stretch of highway many times, in both directions, but couldn't recall ever heading from OKC to Tulsa at dawn, so the view was strange, fresh. Oklahoma City sits at about 1,200 feet above sea level. Tulsa is just below 700 feet, so we were on a slight downhill grade. From every hilltop the low, dark, wooded hills of the ancient, tangled crosstimbers layered out to the smudged horizon, separated by thin strips of summer mist as day flourished in the wings, preparing for its entrance.

There are low, misty, wooded hills everywhere. Why do I love these the most? My father's death had led me to these Oklahoma hills, where I belong, and to the good life I've had here.

Vernon Mack Higgs

When I got the call, in October 1978, that my father had collapsed and was in a coma, and had been rushed from Richmond, Indiana, to a University Hospital in Indianapolis, I'd been living in Portland, Oregon, for about six months. I had no intentions of leaving. I'd become familiar with the bus routes, the city's streets, bridges and parks. I'd found a job as a clerk in the radiology department of a hospital. I'd begun to make connections. I'd had a couple of flings with pretty young women who wore white uniforms at work. When the call came, at work, I hung up the phone, quit my job immediately, strode to the payroll department, and demanded that they write me a check for all due wages on the spot. I don't have any idea how I convinced them to do it. My distress must have been persuasively intimidating because within a short time, as I paced back and forth in front of the receptionist, they'd cut me a check. By the next day, I'd converted it into a one-way airline ticket to Indianapolis and was flying east. My brothers Danny and Mike picked me up from the airport, and we joined our mother, our sister Elaine, and our brother Tim at the hospital. I remember the way we looked at each other, and the way we looked away from each other. Our familiar faces twisted into unfamiliar shapes.

The hospital air seemed pressurized and poisonous. My father was in a darkened ICU ward, tubes running in and out of him. His face was swollen. When I looked at him, I knew that I'd never seen stillness until then. It was terrifying. Someone told me it was okay to talk to him, that I should talk to him, tell him whatever I wanted, because there was no reason to think that he couldn't hear me, just because he couldn't respond. I didn't say much. I told him that I knew he was going to get better. I knew it because we all needed him to get better, and he'd always, without fail, given us what we'd needed. I told him that, and I told him that I loved him.

My father, Vernon Mack Higgs, was born in a cabin on Spade Mountain near Stillwell, Oklahoma, in Cherokee country, on June 7, 1925. A distant relative who still lived in the area took Danny and me to the site once. He showed us the nearby spring where they'd gotten their water, and kept their milk cool. There was no trace left of their home (that we could see) on that shady mountainside. When Dad was nine years old, during the Great Depression, during the Dust Bowl years, his parents, Daniel and Viola, lost their modest claim. They moved to Heber Springs, Arkansas, in the Ozarks, to live with relatives. Within a year or two, his father had died. About that time, probably by no coincidence, his formal education ended with the fourth grade. He was exempted from the draft a few years later, during World War II, because he was "the sole support of his mother." My own mother, Kathleen Elizabeth Adams, first saw him when he was about nineteen. He and another young man stopped into her school one winter's day while they were out rabbit hunting, to warm up by the school stove. She was fourteen. "I never paid him no mind," she told me (sixty-four years later).

He would probably be considered "functionally illiterate" by those who use such terms, but he loved to read, and he loved to read one thing: Louis L'Amour westerns. He always had at least one going at any given time. The only thing I can recall seeing my dad *write* was his signature: V. M. Higgs, in an old-fashioned script. I remember the first time I ever felt protective of him, rather than protected by him. I was about eighteen years old. It was time for him to renew his driver's license. I went with him to the county seat of Greenville, Ohio. The woman behind the counter told him where to sign his new license, and he signed it in his usual way. But then she told him that he would have to sign his whole name, just as she'd typed it. She typed up another one and set it on the counter in front of him and waited. He looked at it for a few seconds, and then looked at me, and with a nod of his head, he beckoned me away from the counter. "I can't remember how to make an r," he said quietly. My heart went out to him. I discreetly showed him how to make an r on a piece of scrap paper.

He and my mother never had a bank account, ever. They came out of the Great Depression, so they didn't trust banks, and they came out of the Ozarks, so they didn't have any money anyway. They had five kids instead. We grew up "rural poor," although he had a steady union job. There were plenty of things we'd have liked more of, under his "sole support," but love

254

was never one of them. His every action and thought, and my mother's, were oriented to taking care of the family. He often couldn't give his children what they wanted, but he always, without fail, gave us what we needed. He was devoted to us, and we to him.

He did not get better. Eight days after he'd gone into a sudden, terrifying fit of pain from a blood vessel bursting in his brain, as he and Mike were working on a car in Mike's front yard, eight days after he'd been knocked off his feet by a blow from within, eight days after I'd been called home, the phone rang at Mom and Dad's house. I remember the six of us, Mom and my siblings and me, shuttling back and forth during those eight cold days, between Richmond and Indianapolis, huddled together in fear, giving the world dirty looks. I happened to answer the phone when it rang. A professional-sounding voice, one of the doctors, advised me that they'd come to the conclusion that my father would not recover—in fact, had not recovered—and was continuing to breathe and pump blood due only to the life-support systems, which they felt they should remove, but they needed permission.

"Go ahead and unhook it." The words came from inside me, but I didn't know the boy who spoke them. After those words had passed from me, I felt emptied of all words forever. I had no more use for words. I hung up the phone. My father was dead. My family was all frozen in place, looking at me. Our father was dead. My mother's husband was dead.

Up until then, whenever someone had asked me to explain who I was, my self-explanation inevitably led to an explanation of who my father was. The only thing I seemed to know for sure, when asked, was that I was my father's son. Now that he was dead, now that I had no father, who was I? It would be years before I could devise an answer.

We had his funeral in Heber Springs, where he and my mother had courted and married. We buried him in a country cemetery several miles out along a winding road east of town. In the family gatherings that followed over the next week, I met two uncles, Bud and Bill, whom I'd mostly known from family photographs. Bud and Bill were my mother's brothers. They lived in Chanute, Kansas, and were in the oil business, which happened to be booming in 1978, due to an OPEC embargo. By the time we'd parted, they'd offered me a job, and I'd accepted.

In The Oil Patch

Two weeks later, a friend drove me across Indiana, Illinois, and Missouri to Kansas, a place I'd never been. I was glad to escape from the grim Indiana November, where the world had become white with grief and black with death, and it grew colder every day. Emerging from rumpled, wooded, and watered Missouri out onto the Kansas plains felt like stepping outside on a brilliant day. I fell instantly in love with the big blue sky and unreachable horizons of the grassy Flint Hills. Oil prices were at record highs, so oilmen were poking holes in every pasture, woodlot, streambed, hilltop, backyard, or ghost town square in that old oil patch between Kansas City and Tulsa. I spent a little over a year riding in trucks with Bill and Bud throughout that area. They were known and liked everywhere. They were kind and patient with me. Those rolling grasslands were especially sweet when spring came, as new green grass sprouted up through last year's tall dead stems from the black gumbo mud. Watery ribbons trickled quietly over exposed limestone hillsides. Moist, fragrant winds blew up from Oklahoma. Some people say that the name Kansas, from the Kansa Indian tribe, refers to "People of the South Wind." When I was there it was the south wind that always blew the sweetest.

We provided two services to the oilmen. First, we logged their wells, which meant we lowered a radioactive pellet of Americium Beryllium to the bottom of the freshly drilled well on a cable, and then drew it back up to the wellhead. The pellet emitted gamma rays out into the strata, and as they bounced back they were picked up by a sensor, as the sensor and pellet were drawn back up at a steady rate. How far the rays penetrated the rock, and how long it took them to bounce back to the sensor, was translated by a pin reader in the back of the truck, similar to a seismograph, thereby creating the log. Petroleum geologists could read these logs because each different stratum has a recognizable pattern. If they thought there might be oil in a particular stratum, or "formation," they could determine from the log precisely how far down that formation was from the wellhead, as well as its porosity and other markers to evaluate the likelihood of its containing oil.

Once the logs were read, we might be directed to perform a second service: perforate the well pipe. We did this by lowering a string of shaped charges we called "shots"–explosive glass balls about the size of tennis balls— down to the desired depth. Packed inside each ball was a metal cone surrounded by explosives. When we detonated the explosives, the force would invert the cones, turning them into powerful bullets that would blow holes through the side of the well pipe. This was how the oil, if they were lucky, could flow from the surrounding stone into the well and then be pumped up to the surface to make everybody rich.

Nobody knows the lay of the land like an experienced oil man. He knows it in three dimensions. He knows the surface, every hill and dale, and he has a clear picture of all the layers below his feet, from the Precambrian basement rock, all the way up to the limestone, sandstone, or shale that he stands on. He knows the names of all the formations and the unvarying order in which they are stacked. He knows about how deep a given formation should be from a given spot on the surface and approximately how thick it should be. He knows where each formation juts to the surface. If he stubs his toe, he knows the name of the rock that did it. And the name of the man who owns the rock. I listened to those oilmen, learning from them just where I stood on the earth.

I lived in Chanute, Kansas, for fourteen months and never made a friend outside the family. I loved and admired Bill and Bud, and got on well with my aunts and cousins, but I was grieving for my father. A deep depression lay below my surface. It isolated me, made me awkward, shy, self-conscious. People could see the strain behind my smile, and it made them keep their distance. Sensing their caution isolated me further. I was no fun at parties. Sometimes my depression gushed to the surface, usually unexpectedly, sometimes embarrassingly. A young woman I'd met invited me once to a pig roast. A team of men had prepared a pig, buried it in a pit of hot coals in the ground, out on the prairie, and took turns tending it for three days and nights. When it was ready, they threw a keg party around the pit. People came from all over. The succulent pig was raised from the pit, as people cheered and gathered around with their drinks. Standing in the midst of men and women whose bloodlines had known each other for generations, I began to shiver. I couldn't stop. The shiver became a quake. I couldn't speak. "Calm down, now, buddy," some guy said to me, but I couldn't. Someone led me away. I suppose it was the woman who'd brought me. I'd wanted so much to join in, but I just couldn't. I was a stranger to myself and others.

Not long before I left Chanute for the bright lights of Tulsa, I came out of a convenience store with some little purchase, and settled in behind the wheel of the old panel truck I'd bought from Bill. I put the key in the ignition. I started the engine. I began to cry. It came from nowhere and over-whelmed me in seconds. I sat there with the engine running, tears soaking my face, sobbing away. People scurried past me, averting their eyes. It went on for three or four minutes. Drained and embarrassed, I drove slowly to the little mobile home I was renting, lay down on my couch, and looked at the ceiling for a long time. I took a shower, as hot as I could stand it, and then hotter still, until I'd drained the hot water heater. After that, I felt a lot better. I knew I had to leave that town.

How I Got to Tulsa

In our oil patch rambles, Bud, Bill and I had had a few occasions to pass through the city of Tulsa. I gawked at its glittering twentieth-century skyline rising above the Arkansas River. Tulsa is a young city, born with the automobile and raised on oil in the booming 1920s. It had been known as the Oil Capital of the World for most of its brief history, until the oil booms moved elsewhere. Then, in the late 1970s and early 1980s, it thrived for a while in a noisy echo of its earlier glory days. I gave Bud and Bill two weeks' notice in December, and moved into an apartment near Riverside Drive, in Tulsa, on January 1, 1980. New month, new year, new decade, new me. I didn't know a soul in the city, including my own. But I was ready to get acquainted.

Most people who arrive in Tulsa, or any city, arrive there first, and over time, perhaps, venture out into the surrounding areas, gradually accruing an understanding of its setting. My experience was the opposite. I've lived in Tulsa for thirty years now and still meet people all the time, some of whom were born and raised there, who have only the vaguest idea of where it is, where they are. Because I'd spent over a year exploring the backroads, small towns, prairies, and woodlands around Tulsa (and beyond) in the hunt for oil, I understood how Tulsa was situated in the landscape long before I entered the city.

I felt at home in Tulsa from the first day. There was something familiar about it, like it was my hometown of Richmond all grown up. The boom was in full swing. The newspapers were loaded with page after page of help wanted ads. The local economy was at odds with the rest of the nation. The embargo had shocked the national economy with a bad recession and inflation. People were suffering from high prices and no work all over the country, outside the oil patch. Since Tulsa's was an oil economy, business was booming, and the population swelled. There were people there from all over the country, and the world, looking for work and looking for business, mixing it up in the jammed saloons. There was (and always had been, and still is) a thriving music scene in town, with some of the best musicians in the world kicking out rock and roll, blues, country, jazz, pop, and various amalgamations every night of the week, all over the place, with no cover charge. Tulsa has been home for me ever since, except for about a year and a half, when I was an over-the-road truck driver.

Home At Last

By the time Joe and I entered the city of Tulsa, in our faithful Land Rover, the sun had risen. Our attempts at conversation had become incoherent. Familiar streets and buildings stuttered past like a DVD on fast forward, skipping every fourth frame. Joe blurted some final navigation suggestions, which were (not unlike "Louie, Louie") unintelligible at any speed. Forcing myself to concentrate, I stopped on red and went on green, used my turn signals, maintained a proper speed, turned in the right places, and pulled safely to a stop in front of my house. It was 6:30 in the morning. We'd driven for 23 hours, 1,200 miles, only stopping for brief rests and supper in Albuquerque. I unloaded my bags, and we stood on the street. I called for a high-five. It came out "hiive," and we missed each other's hands. Our faces cracked in bleary, watery, slit-eyed grins. Joe pulled away as I shouldered my bags one last time and walked up my steps to my own front door. The Oklahoma air was soft, and fragrant from Louise's flower beds. Summer heat was gathering, as were the sounds of a city getting started on its workday.

At the front door I set my bags down, and then remembered that I didn't have my key. Louise wasn't expecting me until the afternoon, and the house was silent and unlit from within, so she was still asleep. I didn't want to wake her by banging on the door, so I sat down on the step to wait, head in hands, until she woke up. As soon as I sat down, I remembered where I'd put the key three weeks before: under the mat. I got back on my feet just as reluctantly as I'd sat down, kicked off my boots, and silently let myself in. I padded through my quiet house like an intruder. My cat darted into another room when she saw me. I knew I couldn't wake Louise without startling her so I opened the bedroom door with care. I watched her sleep for a few seconds before I began to undress. She must have heard my belt buckle because she rose up with a cry, her eyes rolling around for a moment before landing on me. "It's okay," I said quietly. "It's just me. I got home early. We drove all night." I collapsed into bed beside her and closed my eyes.

www.ingramcontent.com/pod-product-compliance
Lightning Source LLC
Chambersburg PA
CBHW072116270326
41931CB00010B/1577